Change Your Mind Change Your Body

How to Have *Permanent Weight-Loss* Success for a More Confident and Happier You!

Wendy Higdon, M.A., LMFT

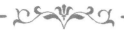

ISBN-13: 978-1535112222

ISBN-10: 1535112220

Read what other people from around the world have to say about *Change Your Mind, Change Your Body:*

"Wake up America and read this book! Get a plan of action now in this little gem of a book and start working on a healthier YOU!"—Lindy S.

"This is a MUST read ... This book is different than any other book on weight loss because this book challenges the thought process behind losing weight. You do not need anything more than this book if you are ready to surpass the superficial quick fixes and get to the core. This is not a "quick fix, take a pill, and hope for the best" hoax. This is the real deal using proven methods from a professional. Thank you for changing my mindset to put me on the path of recovery with specific steps to actually accomplish a permanent change."—Carolyn B., New Zealand

"I loved this book. The author is well-qualified to guide us in the matters of weight loss and changing mindsets. Her personal struggles with weight issues and her experience of being a marriage and family therapist give her greater credibility. It's very inspiring. With the Bonus Journal to keep you motivated along the way, there really are no excuses!"—D. Sutton, Self Healing Coach, Spain

"If you have been struggling with weight and are at your wits end, this book can help you win the mental game! It will get you off the diet roller coaster!"—Susan J., Australia

"This is not a quick fix in prep for a holiday; this is a long-term approach to the changing your attitude towards what we are eating. I for one will be following the author's advice."—Shaun G., Poland

"I'm obese, and it is harder than ever to keep weight off. I struggle with my weight, and finally learned from this awesome book, my MIND has a lot to do with it. It helped me identify belief systems and patterns I wasn't previously aware existed. For the first time in years, I believe I can now succeed at losing and keeping off weight, by following this practical guide."—Nora T.

"I was surprised that this book doesn't stop when you have reached your goal; it continues to guide you through the difficult job of keeping it off."—Julianne B., M.A., LMFT

"Wendy believes she wrote a book to help us lose weight. What she wrote is a book that is far better. She packed this book full of interesting life lessons. Yes, it will put a person who wants to lose weight on the path to do so. In addition, there are deep revelations made possible by this book."—Steven N.

"I can't think of a thing this book doesn't cover! Anyone who's ever been on a 'diet' knows the frustration of struggling through the sacrifices, only to gain the weight back. Wendy Higdon invites the reader to dig down to the core beliefs and experiences that brought us to the place we are today. She leaves no corner unexamined!"—Kim A.

"I was thankful for practical questions, lists, and steps the author gives, while feeling as if she is joining me on my journey."—Ben T.

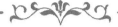

Dedication

To all of you who struggle with your weight,
I dedicate this book to you!

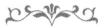

Acknowledgements

I began this writing process not knowing whether I had enough material and ideas to write a whole book. With the help and support of the Self-Publishing School community, I was instructed each step of the way. In the context of this amazing group, we all helped each other to become believers in the process of becoming best-selling authors.

A big shout-out to Chandler Bolt and his team at Self-Publishing School as well as my coach Emily Rose, my accountability partner Nora Truscello, my editor Wayne H. Purdin, my cover designer Heidi Sutherlin, and my formatter Angie Mroczka.

To Dorsey, my wonderful husband, for all his support with help in editing, bigger picture input, and in my being gone on many Saturdays for the completion of this book.

A special shout-out to Kathy Johns, who encouraged me to write what I was passionate about.

To my many friends who encouraged me along the way, indicating they couldn't wait for this book to come out. I am deeply grateful to all of you!

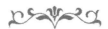

TABLE OF CONTENTS

READ THIS FIRST 11

PREFACE...13

INTRODUCTION...17

THE PROBLEM...21

Chapter 1: How Did We Get To Be This Way? 23

Chapter 2: Am I Really a Food Addict? Here's How to Tell! 35

Chapter 3: Consequences of Our Love of Food 43

Chapter 4: No More Excuses! 49

THE PROCESS 57

Chapter 5: What Are My Pain Points? How Do They Affect My Self Concept?... 59

Chapter 6: Where Does My Change Begin?....................75

Chapter 7: "Stinkin' Thinkin'" (Cognitive Distortions) . 85

Chapter 8: Creating My New Identity 93

Chapter 9: Watch Your Triggers! 101

Chapter 10: Danger Ahead: Watch Out for Sabotage! ..109

Chapter 11: Habits Will Make You or Break You!......... 119

Chapter 12: Accountability: It's Up to Me! 129

THE PLAN **137**

Chapter 13: Where Do I Start?.................................... **139**

Chapter 14: Stress—Do I Need a "Chill Pill"? **153**

Chapter 15: Sleep, Glorious Sleep!............................ **167**

Chapter 16: Exercise—It Really ISN'T the "E" Word **181**

THE PROMISE...**195**

ADDENDUM **199**

ABOUT THE AUTHOR **217**

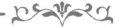

READ THIS FIRST

You will have the most success with this book if you use the journal as you read. You may want to get some friends together to use the journal and provide a support network in your weight-loss success journey.

Just to say thank you for buying my book, I'd like to give you my Change Your Mind, Change Your Body Companion Journal for FREE!

Download the Change Your Mind, Change Your Body Companion Journal at:

http://www.wendyhigdon.com/journal

For further assistance and coaching in your weight-loss journey, visit http://www.wendyhigdon.com

PREFACE

I know you. I've been in your shoes and in your too-tight clothes. I know how you feel about food and the constant struggle with weight. Here's my story.

I began my weight-loss journey long before the age of 11. I was chubby as a kid in the 1950s when no one was overweight, or if they were, they were the rare exception. I often heard my mother say, "That's okay. When she turns 11, I'm going to put her on a diet." In the meantime, there was ample access to goodies—my mom baked cookies, brownies, and cupcakes (even Hostess cupcakes with the filling inside and the squiggle on top) twice a week and kept them in a Tupperware container by the back door as we went out to play. Whole milk was a staple in those days and was delivered directly to your door by the milkman. You could get ice cream delivered at the same time if you wanted. After the evening meal came dessert.

Plenty of tempting foods were everywhere, training my taste buds to relish them. I knew the day would come when all this would go away; a change would be made, not by internally choosing to do so, but by external forces. As a compliant child, I went along with the new program. Fortunately, the girl next door wanted to lose weight before entering high school. She had a tonsillectomy a few months before and gained weight from eating ice cream in her recovery. Armed with a support system and a nutritional plan, we lost our weight and met our goals together. Even as an 11-year-old, I saw how well-meaning people could have sabotaged my efforts if I had listened. "Here, just try a few crumbs of cake," or "You can lick the beaters; it won't hurt you." These were the very people who wanted me to lose weight; yet, if I had given in, they would have sabotaged my efforts.

Over the years, I've had a few ups and downs, but I always came back to my desired weight. It has taken desire, commitment, giving up short-term gratification for long-term benefit, identifying my triggers, and being aware of sabotaging behaviors by others and myself. I learned to counteract all the negative self-talk and berating myself for the shame and disappointment I felt when I failed. After I finally lost weight and internalized my new body image, my behaviors changed so I could maintain the "new me." I had to believe I deserved being more fit, healthier, and happier as a result. I've had 55 years of experience in keeping weight off since that fateful day of my first encounter with weight loss at the age of 11.

❧❧❧

Diets will work. You will lose weight. You know this. You have already tried a number of them and lost weight, but sadly, regained it back and then some.

What happens after a diet that causes you to regain the weight? Do you feel free of the constraints and are ready to enjoy some forbidden foods in moderation? That moderation can lead to the old eating habits that led you there in the first place. This begins the pattern of yo-yo dieting.

I've heard it said many times that one needs to make a lifestyle change after shedding unwanted pounds. We typically think of that in terms of what we eat. I would like to take it a step further to include a lifestyle of changing our mindset about food and how we see ourselves in order to maintain our new image. Imagine your slim self, full of energy and confidence. Then ask yourself, "What will I need to do to maintain the new me?"

My intention is that this book and journal will be a trusted guide and companion to whatever diet efforts you choose to pursue. The success or failure of diet plans is in the implementation of them. That's the thrust of this book—to help you with a mindset change and tools to navigate your way through the bumpy waters in such an undertaking. Losing weight and keeping it off is hard work, but you can do this!

If you're eager to get started on your journey of losing weight, you can jump ahead to Chapter 13 to learn about personality differences, how to understand yourself a little better, and how it might affect which eating plan you choose. You will need to do your own research on the best diet plan for you. I've listed a few to get you started; you may already have one that has worked for you in the past. The important thing is that you embrace one you believe you can be successful with. Believing you can do this is a key component to your success.

Now let's get started!

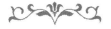

INTRODUCTION

Stress—we face it more or less every day with broken relationships, dysfunctional families, disappointments, and demands of balancing job and family life. It's easy to comfort ourselves with food when we're stressed. Has turning to food been a lifelong pattern of temporarily relieving stress and emotional pain?

Can you identify with any of the following scenarios?

When going to an office party or potluck with lots of goodies, Christine wants to "be good" but ends up eating too much. She later feels guilty and berates herself for it. This was supposed to be a time to enjoy conversations with others, yet she comes away feeling depressed and defeated.

Robert falls into the trap of eating something he shouldn't; he then plays the same old broken record of negative self-talk, magnifying his weaknesses and minimizing his strengths.

Frances finds herself mindlessly eating because she's bored or lonely and later feels like a failure for not finding better ways to be in control of her life.

If these sound familiar, are you tired of these never-ending scenarios of pain in your life—feeling disgust, shame, guilt, and regret? When will you say, "Enough is enough"? Are you ready to face patterns and behaviors that keep you stuck in your present struggles with food?

While the market is full of books on dieting and weight loss, my intent in *Change Your Mind, Change Your Body* is to help you navigate your weight-loss efforts to create a new healthy lifestyle. This book looks at the basic patterns and belief systems that hold you back from living an energized and happier life without all the blaming and shaming.

Change Your Mind, Change Your Body gives you insights into managing your relationship with food in a more productive way. This book is a readable guide to help you overcome your resistance, develop new beliefs, and empower yourself to reclaim your life. It also provides practical guidelines, including how to visualize the "new you" to set you up for success. If you're tired of repeating the same bad eating patterns that wreak havoc on your emotions and you're ready to make changes, this book is for you.

Why should you want to listen to me? I've struggled with weight issues since the age of 11 and have been successful at keeping weight off for 55 years. Along the way, I've had ups and downs, needing to lose a few pounds here and there. I'm also a licensed marriage and family therapist. I understand human behaviors and negative belief systems that get in our way, and I have helped many to make changes in their lives.

Through reading *Change Your Mind, Change Your Body*, you will identify your resistance to changing eating habits, what's keeping you stuck with self-sabotaging behaviors, and how to live your life to be successful in your weight-loss journey.

Let this book help you change longstanding behaviors that sabotage your efforts to take control of your life. It's time to make those changes, and this book can help you do just that!

If you take the time to reflect on how you've kept yourself mired down in your struggles with your weight and your relationship with food, you can change what you're willing to acknowledge.

Isn't it time to stop this never-ending cycle of disgust, self-hatred, and frustration with your weight issues and relationship with food? Aren't you ready to see a new day with happiness, confidence, and contentment? Isn't it time?

It's not selfish to take care of yourself. If you don't, you can't take care of others. Your families, friends, and work suffer. When on an aircraft, the flight attendant instructs adult passengers to put on the oxygen mask first in order to help their children. If the adults pass out, they no longer can help anyone. Therefore, focusing on making yourself your #1 priority is not selfish; it's the beginning of being happier and more productive in the service of others.

I promise you that if you follow this easy-to-read guide, you will identify what's holding you back and reclaim yourself as priority #1. Don't miss out on gaining mastery over your struggles with food. Be the role model that your family and others will be inspired by. They will wonder, "I don't know how she/he does that," and they will want what you have. It's time to be healthy and to have more energy for you, your family, and social events. It's time to take *action now* and conquer your weight struggles once and for all!

In this book, you will find the concepts of how to break bad habits of overeating as I did.

I am including a free journal for you to download and use as you read this book. You will find references to the journal in italics in the book. It's important to do the exercises as you make lifelong change. The temptation is to keep reading. DON'T! Do the exercises! The concepts and applications of changing lifelong sabotaging thoughts and behaviors will propel you to conquer your weight-loss struggles.

Thank you for trusting me to share this journey with you. Losing weight is hard work; it's even harder to come to terms with the need and desire to shed those pounds. Admitting your problem and deciding to do something about it is 90% of the battle won; you're on your way. You're now taking control of your life and putting yourself at the top of your list. This is your time to make a change to enjoy the new life you're meant to live. Watch yourself transform before your very eyes. It's time. It's way past time! The road ahead will bring challenges and hard work, but when you cross that finish line, you will rejoice and know that the journey was well worth it. It's time to begin!

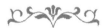

THE PROBLEM

Chapter 1:
How Did We Get To Be This Way?

"Houston, we [have] a problem."
—Astronaut John Swigert, Jr., Apollo 13

America ... the overweight society. How did we become so overweight with two-thirds of the American population being classified as overweight or obese? It hasn't always been this way. Do you remember watching *Leave It to Beaver* or seeing reruns? Do you remember Lumpy? He was considered fat and was made

Growing up as a child, I was chubby in a world that wasn't.

fun of because of his weight. If you were to transpose him into today's society, he would fit right in and wouldn't be considered to have a weight problem at all; well, maybe he could lose a few, but he's really "okay."

I was the female version of Lumpy in the 1950s. Growing up as a child, I was chubby in a world that wasn't. Although bullying hadn't become as pronounced as it is today, there was still a stigma against being overweight. I felt it every day because I knew deep down inside that I wasn't "as good as" my friends. At home, when I finally went on my first diet at the age of 11, it was clear that the rules were different for me.

My brothers drank whole milk whereas I was given skim milk, which tasted like water compared to the fat-laden whole milk I was accustomed to. No more treats going out the back door to play. A new day of looking at food had begun.

So how did we become so overweight? Sugar has certainly played a role in this. Let's take a short side trip to learn about the evolution of sugar, as we know it today.

Origins of Sugar and Food Addiction

The following history of sugar was outlined by Rich Cohen in a recent article in National Geographic Magazine.[1] In New Guinea, people ate sugar cane raw and continued chewing it until they hit the "sweet spot," creating pleasure when dopamine levels rise. Sugar came to the Asian continent in 1000 B.C. and was refined as a powder in 500 A.D. in India. It spread to Persia and followed Islam wherever the Koran was taught, according to Sidney Mintz, author of *Sweetness and Power*.

It eventually was introduced to Britain and France from the Crusades and was available to only the nobility. From there it made its way to the Atlantic Islands, and Christopher Columbus brought it to the New World on his second voyage. Soon the Caribbean Islands were filled with sugar cane plantations and slavery to provide for increased consumption. Prices fell and demand went up, making sugar a staple for the middle class and the poor.

Our Love of Sugar

Over time, we've consumed more and more sugar. In 1700, the British consumed four pounds of sugar per person in a year; by 1800, the numbers rose to 18 pounds of sugar; and in 1870, they ate 47 pounds of sugar per person. We're still not satisfied. By 1900, the average Englishman now consumed 100 pounds annually. The average American takes in 77 pounds of added sugar each year, which equals 22 teaspoons of sugar a day.

Richard Johnson, a nephrologist at the University of Colorado in Denver, wanted to know why only five percent of the world's population had high blood pressure in 1900, yet one-third of the population now has high blood pressure. What about the 153 million people with diabetes in 1980? Now, there are 347 million

Sugar is like a poison and is toxic in high doses...

worldwide, more than double in 30 years. Sugar is believed to be the major culprit with studies showing high amounts of sugar in our diets. This has led to high levels of fat and insulin in our bloodstream, leading to heart disease and diabetes.

Sugar as a Drug

Sugar is like a poison and is toxic in high doses, according to endocrinologist Robert Lustig of the University of California, San Francisco.[1] The obvious answer to this dilemma is to decrease our consumption of sugar! When we do, many of the resulting ill effects will resolve themselves. We may not be able to avoid all sugar, but we can certainly cut back.

How are we so drawn in by sugar? Why did it become a delicacy and follow the development of civilizations? Sugar is not classified as a drug; it's legal, and we all love it. But why do we love it so much? What causes us to crave the food we know isn't good for us? When we give in to our cravings, it causes an increase in dopamine (our brain's pleasure center), and we experience pleasure. Eventually, dopamine levels decrease, according to Dr. Susan Peirce Thompson, former Professor at Monroe Community College in Rochester, New York, and the cravings return.[2]

She describes the comparison of sugar and flour to cocaine

Sugar ... brings pleasure; when we stop eating it, depression, fatigue, and irritability take over, and we crash.

and heroin and the effect it has on the brain. Let's look at the manufacturing of cocaine and heroin to make a link. Cocaine is produced from the coca leaf which, in and of itself, is harmless. When the coca leaf is refined into a powder, it becomes a drug that's addictive.

The same is true for heroin. Heroin is made from poppies. By themselves, poppies aren't harmful; we use poppy seeds in cooking and baking. When the poppy plant is refined into a fine powder, known as heroin, it also becomes addictive.

Sugar follows suit. We can make sugar from corn, beets, or sugar cane. There is nothing wrong with those foods. Corn on the cob is often a staple at a summertime barbecue. When we take these foods and refine them into powder, into sugar, it becomes addicting, just as cocaine and heroin are. Sugar increases our dopamine levels and brings pleasure; when we stop eating it, depression, fatigue, and irritability take over, and we crash. We eat more to feel better again. We get away with it because sugar is legal, and cocaine and heroin are not. Did you know that rats prefer sugar to cocaine? They become addicted to the sweet taste, which hooks their brains into wanting more.

The same can be said for flour. Whether it's made from wheat, rice, barley, oats, or other grains, the process of refining it into a powder gives us a product that turns a natural grain into a drug.[2]

Turn to page 6 in your journal. Think about how sugar and flour affect how you feel and function.

What has happened from the 1950s when we had access to sugar, but most of America wasn't overweight? Many women were home, raising children and preparing home-cooked meals, and dinnertime was honored and a way to reconnect with family. With fast-food restaurants springing up in the late 1950s and 1960s, we began to enjoy easy access to good-tasting food whenever we wanted. As more women joined the work force, the convenience of fast food made its way into our lives as a staple.

Is it any wonder that we live in a food-addicted society? With the arrival of good-tasting food to comfort us and lull us into a daze, dulled by oblivion and nonfunctioning, we've given in to the temptations all around us, and there are plenty of them. Everywhere we go, we see commercials or billboards for tantalizing foods. What about burgers that drip with flavor and fat? Or advertisements for ice cream and other sweets? They call you in for business to take a buck or more from you, but they do nothing for your health and well-being; it's only a fix for the moment, a way to medicate your pain and soothe your frazzled nerves for a short time. You may be hungry, but a quick drive-through doesn't help your overall health when you do it over and over. Then it's back to reality.

Even kids are lured by cereal commercials, which is a mother's nightmare while shopping for groceries with her kids. She hears, "Mom! Can I have that cereal?" Another child says, "No, I want this one." A third chimes in, "No, this is the one I want." The harassed mother has to deal with three temper tantrums at once, needing to leave the store and return later without meltdowns from junk food marketing. We have given in to these temptations over and over, and it shows on our bodies, our demeanor, our energy levels, and our health.

There are consequences to our poor eating habits and food addictions. Our bodies are meant to be well-oiled machines. Extra body fat reduces our life span, and the extra weight drains our energy. About one in five American deaths each year are related to obesity. It is the second leading preventable cause of death behind tobacco use. Each year approximately 300,000 people DIE as a result of conditions related to obesity,

That's about 100 World Trade Centers every year. Where's the outcry? Where's the rage?

according to the National Institutes of Health.[3] That's about 100 World Trade Centers every year. Where's the outcry? Where's the rage? This isn't an attack by terrorists from the outside; we're doing this to ourselves. We're complacent with an apathetic attitude, and it doesn't even faze us.

Even though we have been brainwashed and seduced into eating sugar and unhealthy foods, we're still responsible to make changes in our eating for better health, more energy, and greater happiness.

Causes of Obesity

What causes obesity? Probably the biggest factor in our obesity dilemma is food addiction. There are several reasons people are overweight besides food addiction. Genetics can play a part, but usually it's caused by eating more calories than are being burned.[4] If you have a slow metabolism, you have to work harder at losing and maintaining weight and doing things to increase your metabolism. Working with a nutritionist or a holistic doctor can help you fine-tune what will work for you.

Probably the biggest factor in our obesity dilemma is food addiction.

Medical Causes

There are medical conditions that cause weight gain. Before starting any weight-loss program of lifestyle change and exercise, you should get a good physical from your doctor to rule out any medical concerns and to give you a green light for exercise. Hypothyroidism can lead to a slowed metabolism, which can contribute to weight gain, and it can be an underlying source of depression. Other neurological problems make weight management difficult, so it's best to work with your doctor.

With more people taking psychotropic medications, the increased use of these medications has contributed to obesity. Weight gain can be a side effect. If this is happening to you, ask your doctor if there is another medication that will not cause weight gain. There are options to manage your condition and minimize the side effects. Talk with your doctor about your options.

Psychological Causes

Psychologically, we use food to comfort ourselves, whether it's to calm our anxiety or to relieve stress. If we're sad, have a bad day, or simply don't feel good about ourselves, we turn to food for comfort. We lose ourselves for the moment in the pleasure we get from eating something that tastes good. In that moment, our pain is gone. We call this "self-medicating." Just as alcoholics and drug addicts "medicate their pain," we do the same thing with food. Our medicating with food is, to a lesser degree, avoidance of dealing with pain. It is a temporary fix that can create new problems all of their own (loss of health and loss of self-worth).

When we overeat, we often have regrets, self-hatred, fall into a depressed mood, feel disgusted, and may even continue to overeat to medicate these feelings. As in any addiction, we must go back to the problems we're avoiding, even if it's something as simple as avoiding stress or boredom. Overeating doesn't necessarily need to be defined as an addiction; when we lose sight of making better choices to deal with our frustrations, anger, stress, anxiety, and depression, we need to look at better coping strategies to manage our emotions instead of resorting to the comfort of food.

If you're a food addict, you cannot escape eating. We need food to live, it's less expensive than drugs, and it's available everywhere. Family, friends, and our culture push food on us 365 days a year. We become obese, and others don't realize we're addicted to food. They don't see our pain being medicated by food; instead, they may see us as being unmotivated and lazy.

Weight-loss programs, for the most part, don't deal with food addiction and give only superficial solutions. With two-thirds of Americans being overweight or obese, we're in denial about our addictions and habits of overeating.

Environmental Causes

Environmental causes of being overweight are probably the biggest factor of all. The good news is that we can do something about it. And that IS good news!

Food is everywhere. We need it to live, to sustain life; everywhere we turn, it somehow shows up. It shows up at work—candy on someone's desk, donuts and coffee at break time, office meetings with catered food, potlucks, vending machines, and even our own desk drawer.

What about the drive to work or the drive home after a long day of work and stress? What kind of billboards do you see? Advertisements for fat-laden juicy burgers with fries and a soft drink, Dunkin Donuts, and anything that would make your cares go away are everywhere. You may have your own favorite guilty pleasure, luring you after a hard day at the office. What kinds of eating establishments do you see on your way to and from work? There are McDonald's everywhere (even around the world—my first day in Beirut, Lebanon, there it was, a familiar comfort from home), Burger King, Jack-in-the-Box, Carl's Jr., bakeries, donut shops, ad nauseam, but the lure is for that feed-my-emotions supersized cheeseburger and fries or sweets without end. We don't realize we're being enticed and lured in until the food is gone, and we wonder what we have just done.

What about our kitchens? This is where the majority of our eating comes from unless we can afford to eat out regularly, which comes with a price other than dollars. At home, we have easy access to food. We're tired from work, so we throw in a pizza or snack on chips and salsa. What could be easier than microwave dinners? There are canned foods of pasta, SPAM, packaged foods, such as mac 'n cheese, processed meats, hotdogs, corn dogs, and more frozen foods of ready-made taquitos, burritos, and enchiladas. This is not to mention the high levels of sodium and preservatives, all for our convenience.

With our busy lifestyles, we're neglecting our health for the sake of convenience. This will come with a price for our long-term well-being in health and energy and financial costs with trips to the doctor. What would it mean if we could sacrifice some leisure time to put in the work of healthy meal planning and preparation to take care of ourselves, to be fit and ultimately have more energy and be happier? It takes work to have long-term results vs. giving in to short-term gratification. This includes what we eat, whether or not we exercise, and the priorities we set. We're so busy. Have we taken the time to think about what we want? If we will do that, we can make changes.

With our busy lifestyles, we're neglecting our health for the sake of convenience.

Out go the crackers, the candy, the cookies, the processed and packaged foods, chips, and ice cream. In comes the nutrition that fuels your body and reenergizes you. It naturally helps you to lose those stubborn pounds you continually lug around and don't do anything about. Now you *are* doing something about it. We're talking about leafy greens, vibrant vegetables and fruits, protein, dairy, beans of all kinds, and complex carbohydrates. If you go vegan, there are books and recipes you can enjoy.

You can delight in foods that are good for you and your body. Foods that once were shunned in favor of the easy burger and fries will have new meaning and flavor and will be life-giving as you begin to see the pounds drop off while having more energy.

Turn to page 6 in your journal. Consider the causes of weight gain in your life. Is it from medical, psychological, environmental causes, or a combination of them?

Possible Case Studies

What happens if we continue to comfort ourselves with food and don't deal with our bad eating patterns? If we allow ourselves to keep eating and not exercising, we become obese. It doesn't take much these days. Next time you're at the mall, look around and see overweight people everywhere. This is a sad state of affairs. We're killing ourselves with food. So what are the consequences?

Here are some examples of what this might look like. See if you can relate or you know someone in any of these or similar situations:

1. Susan, age 42, is 120 pounds overweight. She's a single mom with two children, ages 5 and 3, and she has no energy to keep up with them.

2. Victor, 45, was told by his doctor that he needed to lose at least 100 or more pounds, or he could die of a heart attack in the next five to ten years.

3. Valerie, 28, is a beautiful woman having excess weight of nearly 100 pounds. She was sexually assaulted as a teenager and is using her weight to keep men away.

4. Mary found out she has diabetes. She needs to lose about 140 pounds and is now serious to do so.

5. Linda just found out her son, who is in the fifth grade and weighs about double what he should, is having behavior problems as a result of being teased and bullied.

6. James, in his early 20s, is concerned about his parents who are in their 50s and are both about 130 pounds overweight. He wants to know what he can do to help them see that they're in danger of having life-threatening diseases prematurely.

7. Samuel has been depressed for a number of years. He comes from a family that's overweight, and he himself is about 100 pounds overweight. He hasn't considered that his being overweight may be a factor in his depression.

Even though we've been brainwashed and seduced into eating sugar and unhealthy foods, we're still responsible for making changes in our eating for better health, more energy, and greater happiness.

In the next chapter, we will look at food addiction, the signs, and how to tell if you're a food addict. Let's look and see ...

Chapter 2:
Am I Really a Food Addict?
Here's How to Tell!

"Insanity is doing the same thing, over and over again,
but expecting different results."
—Narcotics Anonymous

"I'm not a food addict! I love my food, but I'm not an addict. That's for alcoholics and druggies." Let's look at what food addiction is and see where we stand.

We need food to survive. We can't say, "I'm not going to eat." We have to eat.

Along with survival, we're also gratified with pleasure from food's taste, texture, and aroma. For some people, food can become addictive, just as drugs and alcohol are. Foods high in sugar, fats, and/or salt trigger chemical reactions in our brains, resulting in feeling pleasure and being satisfied. It's the same reward center of the brain that keeps the drug user and alcoholic wanting more.

You become dependent on feeling good from food and want to continue eating. This can cause you to overeat when you're not hungry. You depend on food to give you feelings of well-being rather than finding it in more productive ways. This generates a cycle of overeating to create those pleasurable feelings, beyond what's necessary to feel full. This can lead to physical, emotional, and social consequences, which will be discussed in Chapter 3. Even with these consequences, the food addict finds comfort in food, often being in denial of its effect on his/her life.

Besides the addicting nature of sugar, several other factors can come into play. One is the biological nature of food addiction where there may be a hormonal imbalance, side effects from medications, or having a family history of food addiction.

Another cause of food addiction is from psychological factors, which can include past emotional or sexual abuse, being a victim of trauma, not having coping skills to deal with negative situations, low self-esteem, or going through grief and loss. We resort to food to "medicate" our unpleasant emotions. It's important to find non-food-related coping skills instead to respond to the cues to manage our emotions without food being the vehicle.

You become dependent on feeling good from food and want to continue eating.

There can be social reasons that result in food addiction. These include dysfunction in the family or with friends, pressure from peers or family to eat more than you should ("one more piece of pie won't hurt you"), social isolation, lack of social support, and stressful situations.

How can you tell if you have a food addiction? Here are possible signs or symptoms you may experience:

- eating more food than you intended and making yourself sick

- going out of your way to get a desired food or going for a midnight run

- continuing to eat when you're not hungry anymore

- intentionally eating by yourself

- avoiding social events to spend time eating what you want

- decreased efficiency at work

- spending a lot of time and money on food for bingeing purposes

Some physical symptoms can include:

- chronic fatigue and low energy

- sleep disorders, such as sleep apnea, insomnia, or oversleeping

- being restless

- being more irritable

- headaches or digestive problems

In the field of psychology, there are guidelines to determine whether a person has a problem with drugs or alcohol. I have adapted the criteria from the American Psychiatric Association: Diagnostic and Statistical Manual of Mental Disorders (5th ed.) or DSM-5[1], to get a better look at the impact of food addiction. (This doesn't imply their endorsement; it's my adaptation to addiction criteria.)

Is there a problematic pattern of overeating causing a lot of distress or negative consequences with the following signs or symptoms?

1. You often eat more food and for longer periods than you planned to.

2. You want to cut down the amount you eat and have not been successful to control your eating.

3. A lot of time is spent thinking about food at the expense of optimal functioning.

4. A lot of time is spent in getting food, eating a lot of food, or recovering from its effects (not sleeping well and/or needing to recover the next day).

5. A strong desire or actual craving to eat certain foods.

6. Recurrent overeating, which affects your functioning at work, school, or home.

7. Continued overeating despite negative impact on social or interpersonal problems.

8. You give up important social, work, or recreational opportunities because of your overeating.

9. You continue to overeat when there are physical consequences.

10. You continue to overeat when you know you have a recurrent physical or psychological problem that was caused by or made worse by your overeating, and you don't stop.

11. Tolerance:

    a. You need more food to get your desired effect.

    b. You get less of an effect with the same amount of food.

12. Withdrawal: You have side effects of lethargy and irritability when the food runs its course, and you need more foods with sugar to feel better again.

If you have two or three symptoms from the above list, you probably have a mild food addiction. A moderate addiction would include four or five symptoms, and having six or more means you probably have a severe food addiction. The higher the number, the stricter you need to be with what you eat.

Think of it this way. If you're an alcoholic, you would no longer be able to drink without it taking you where you don't want to go. If you're a food addict, it doesn't take much to lead you down the path of bingeing and overeating. It's just like the Lay's potato chip commercial says, "No one can eat just one."

A legal term, called the bright line rule, is a defined rule or standard, made up of objective factors, which doesn't leave room for varying degrees of interpretation. Its purpose is to ensure predictable and consistent results.

In contrast to bright line rules, there are balancing tests (or "fine line" tests) where several factors are weighed. This makes inconsistencies possible in applying the law, and it can decrease objectivity in making decisions.

In Alcoholics Anonymous, the standard is no drinking. A bright line has been drawn. Sobriety is the standard. The same is true for Narcotics Anonymous. But we have to eat.

Can we apply this concept to our eating habits? Absolutely. We're all different in what we can handle. We can set up our own bright lines. For instance, if we have a weakness for candy, we draw the line to not eat it or have it in the house. Others may be able to have one or two pieces without it sending them into binge eating.

If we use drinking as an analogy, some people can have a drink without a problem. Others often find it difficult to have just one drink and may have three or four or more, giving them a hangover the next day. To take it even further, there are those who are true alcoholics, and one drink leads them into oblivion, down a path of no return. We have to decide how much we can handle and where we have to draw our bright line.

Turn to page 7 in your journal and honestly evaluate yourself from my adapted version of the DSM-5. How many symptoms can you relate to?

Evaluate your eating in light of this. Are you the kind of person who can have an occasional treat and not have it negatively impact your eating habits? Or do you eat more than you planned, and then you have to work through your body digesting all the extra heavy food? Are you addicted to sugar and flour and that is how you eat every day, packing on the pounds?

It's important to understand how you respond to food and the impact it has on you. When you know this about yourself, you can establish your own "bright lines," according to your own response to the addictive nature of sugar. If you have lower numbers, you may be able to eat in moderation. If you are at the extreme end, you will do well to eliminate flour and sugar completely. Check out the resource of Bright Line Eating in Chapter 13.

The numbers you came up with earlier in the chapter will help you determine which eating plan from Chapter 13 resources will be a good fit. The lower the number, the more flexibility you have. The higher the number, the more you will need to eliminate sugar and flour.

Whatever the results are, I hope you have been honest in evaluating your behaviors. There's no judgment; it's important to see where you stand to make necessary changes. This will be helpful information to know when you begin to make plans (Chapter 13) to create a lifestyle change you can live with.

In the next chapter, we will look at the consequences of our overeating and the impact it has on us physically, emotionally, and socially. We must understand "the why" of needing to change our eating patterns, so please keep reading ...

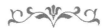

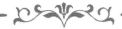

Chapter 3:
Consequences of Our Love of Food

"If you know the 'WHY,' if you really, really know it...
the 'HOW' will always come."
—Mitch Matthews, *The Coach Mindset*

People in different cultures around the world connect socially with each other in sharing food together. And how we enjoy our food and all the pleasures that come with eating and socializing! If we are not careful about the food choices we make when socializing, it's easy to fall into habits of unhealthy eating, leading to consequences from our poor choices and food addictions.

As we saw in Chapter 1, we are killing ourselves with food. The number of people dying every year from preventable causes doesn't even faze us. Are we that much in denial that we don't see we have a problem? Are we that addicted to food that we keep eating the wrong foods and packing on the pounds to our detriment (one of the hallmark signs of addiction)? When will we wake up to see the devastation and destruction we are causing in our own lives and the collateral damage in the lives of others?

I wonder if we consider the amount and kinds of foods we eat that cause us problems. Isn't it a part of American life that we enjoy so much? But our way of life is killing us!

Physical Consequences

Let's look at the physical consequences of our lifestyle we have rationalized for ourselves. The following list has been attributed to our lifestyle of overeating and not exercising:

- Heart disease
- Diabetes
- Hypertension
- Orthopedic problems
- Gallbladder disease
- Osteoarthritis
- Some cancers (uterine, breast, colorectal, kidney, and gallbladder)
- Asthma
- Sleep disorders, such as sleep apnea, which can be fatal
- Pregnancy complications
- High blood cholesterol
- Menstrual irregularities
- Psychological disorders
- Increased surgical risk
- Social discrimination[1]

Let's look into this further.

Heart disease is the leading cause of death in women. A contributing factor is obesity and poor eating habits. There is also diabetes from obesity, which can result in many serious problems. These include kidney failure, stroke, amputation, blindness (#1 cause), cardiovascular disease (two to four times more likely), impotence, and neuropathy (pain and numbness in our extremities). Obesity can also contribute to liver disease, gout, pulmonary problems, and reproductive problems in women, keeping them from conceiving until shedding the pounds.

This is serious business—don't gloss over the list of ailments you may face from becoming obese. Think about each one. What if your doctor told you to lose 50-100 pounds or more to avoid these diseases? If any of these ailments strike you, it is no longer a statistic, but it now becomes *your* reality. Is that what you want? I hope not! Think about this BEFORE you get the words you don't want to hear.

Think about this BEFORE you get the words you don't want to hear.

Besides the above diseases, we can experience the following:

- Decreased energy and fatigue
- Difficulty concentrating
- Patterns of insomnia or oversleeping
- Feeling restless
- Being irritable

Psychological Consequences

Let's look at the damage being done to us psychologically:

Are you depressed and down on yourself because you are overweight? Are you consumed by your thoughts around food? How much time do you spend in negative self-talk, shaming yourself for eating this or that? Have there been times when you've felt disgusted with yourself, and this happens over and over?

We get stuck in these negative loops and have to force ourselves to break out of them. How much time do you think about food in planning what you will eat or going to parties and feeling guilty and disappointed for eating too much of the calorie-laden food? How much time do you spend thinking about your weight—what to wear, what you look like to other people ("Do I look fat in this?")? Do you feel self-conscious at social gatherings and compare yourself to others? You probably think about food and your weight much more than you realize.

Social Consequences

Food addiction can also affect your social life and your relationships:

- Decreased performance at work or at school
- Isolating from family and friends
- Conflicts with family about weight and overeating
- Losing pleasure in doing things you used to enjoy doing

- Avoiding social events
- Putting your finances or career at risk

Go to page 9 in your journal. Take time to jot down how your thoughts about your weight and food are keeping you from optimal functioning in these three areas. Do you have any medical issues that need addressing? Are you fatigued and tired all the time? Are you distracted at work, not focused, not listening in meetings because you're thinking about your weight? How does it affect your social life and your relationships with your spouse, friends, or children?

Benefits of Losing Weight

We have looked at the consequences of our poor eating habits. What if we could conquer our food addictions and become healthy and fit? What would those benefits look like? Here are a few:

- having less stress
- having more energy
- having increased self-esteem
- being more sociable
- being more involved with loved ones, children
- being happier
- having less negative self-talk
- having less physical pain—back, knees, legs
- having better health
- decreasing our chances of life-threatening diseases
- having more peace

- having less worry
- having less irritability
- being more engaged with others
- being less reactive
- being more present
- being more content
- having increased self-worth (tied to body image)

On page 10 in your journal, use the above list of benefits as a starting point to create your list of whys. This will be your motivation and driving force to help you to be successful in your weight-loss efforts.

Isn't it a shame to let food, which is meant for our well-being, take over our lives in negative consequences and keep us from experiencing a better life? Isn't it time to put food in its place and for us to begin to live the lives we were meant to live? It's time to experience the benefits of being healthy and fit!

In the next chapter, we will look at our excuses and how we let ourselves off the hook by rationalizing. In the process, we remain stuck. Let's end our excuses, take responsibility, and have success in managing our weight to create the life we desire to have.

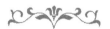

Chapter 4:
No More Excuses!

"Essentially there are two actions in life: performance and excuses. Make a decision as to which you will accept from yourself."—Steven Brown

Excuses! Excuses! We all have them. Why do we allow excuses to take over and sabotage our dreams of being healthy and fit, energized, and happy? Do we accept the status quo to be comfortable? Maybe *too* comfortable. We give in to foods that taste good and soothe our frazzled emotions. Are we subconsciously staying in a rut because we accept the status quo and give up on being anything better? In other words, we settle.

It is time to say, "No more excuses!" It is time to claim our new destiny and the life we desire to have for the rest of our lives. As Roberto Hernandez, winner of *The Biggest Loser, Season 17,* passionately stated after a weigh-in, "We are the fattest country in this world. And this is to you, America. If you just get up, if you just get up from that damn couch and walk a little bit; then the next week you're jogging. America, you can do it. I know there's someone out there, and I know I'm motivating you because I sat on that damn couch, and I saw my little boys play by themselves. They didn't have a father because I was so fat. Let's stop doing this to ourselves and work hard."

We rationalize to make excuses for our behavior to justify our actions. *Merriam-Webster's Dictionary* defines *rationalize* as, "to bring into accord with reason or cause something to seem reasonable: as to attribute (one's actions) to rational and creditable motives without analysis of true and especially unconscious motives ... and to provide plausible but untrue reasons for conduct."[1] Think of the word rationalize as "rational" lies. This is what we tell ourselves—reasonable lies to justify our actions, to give ourselves permission to do what we have second thoughts about doing. We make our behavior "acceptable" when it really ends up sabotaging what we desire for ourselves.

Think of the word rationalize as "rational" lies.

How do we overcome these rational lies we tell ourselves? First, we must catch ourselves doing it. They are insidious— these lies we fall into and then later regret. We rationalize in many ways, not just with food. What are some ways you rationalize?

Stop here and think of the rationalizations (rational lies) you use to make it okay to engage in behavior you know won't be good for you in the long run. Go to page 11 in your journal to record your answers.

Rationalization: "I haven't had this food in such a long time, and I can start back on my eating plan tomorrow."

Consequence: You eat too much because it's so good. You cannot go to sleep because you're too full, and you don't sleep well because your body is digesting the food. You're tired the next day, and you have paid for your indulgence.

Make your list. Keep adding to it as you become aware of more. As part of the consequences, you not only face negative physical results, but also negative emotions, such as disgust, self-hatred, guilt, and the negative self-talk that goes along with these emotions: "I'm such a failure," "I can't do anything right," "When will I ever grow up," "I'm so weak-willed," "I knew better, but I did it anyway," and the negative thoughts keep coming. Add these negative emotions and negative self-talk to your list.

Why is it important to make these lists? When you recognize the traps you set for yourself by rationalization, you will catch yourself and choose another behavior. When you're aware of the possible pitfalls, you can preplan an exit strategy. Now's the time to identify your rationalizations and the consequences you've experienced. While you're working on this, feel the pain caused by giving in to these rational lies. At the time, it made sense to you, but if you took a minute to think about it, you might have chosen differently.

...feel the pain caused by giving in to these rational lies.

Have you become lulled into a sense of complacency? "It's too much work to think of changing, and I'm tired," you tell yourself. "I'm not that bad off. I can start when there's a break in all this work (or when the kids go back to school or leave home or whatever)." You've become desensitized to your need and desire to be healthy, energetic, and happier. Are you settling for less than your best self?

The word *desensitize* is defined as "1) to make an individual insensitive or nonreactive to a sensitizing agent and 2) to make someone emotionally insensitive or callous."[2] This means you extinguish an emotional response (fear, anxiety, or guilt) to stimuli that formerly brought it on.

You're well aware of how TV programs and movies have gradually added sex and violence in small increments, and we're desensitized to it. In order to get a reaction, the moviemakers keep pressing the envelope because we've become used to and tolerate murders and all sorts of violence.

Look at what's happening in today's world. Having school lockdowns is now not out of the ordinary. School shootings don't raise the same horror as they first did with Columbine and Sandy Hook. Half a century ago, this was not even fathomable in our thinking. Students were in trouble for throwing spitballs and chewing gum in class. Now they're killing each other. In listening to the news, we hear of murders, kidnappings, sexual assault as common fare; it no longer horrifies us, and we take it in as the usual news story.

If you want to kill a frog in a pot of hot water, you gradually increase the temperature so he becomes used to it. Eventually he dies (or so the story goes). If you put another frog right into boiling water, he jumps out. He hasn't been desensitized, and his body reacts in self-preservation.

Where is our self-preservation? Have we done the same thing with our weight in being desensitized? What once would have appalled us we now accept. It no longer brings a reaction. We've settled for the status quo; we fit in and we're happy, or so we think.

Claudia Svartefoss writes in her book, *Positively Perfect*, the desensitizing tool is "a quality of our mind that subconsciously adapts us—it desensitizes us to our existing environment. By existing environment we mean our physical environment, but also our non-physical environment of thoughts, beliefs, ideas, opinions, perspectives, preferences, desires, intentions, expectations, interests, and emotions." We get used to feeling the negative emotion because we're desensitized, and we can become complacent with our negative thoughts. She goes on to say "our desensitizing tool usually makes it easier for us to get used to where we are because doing so provides us with the fastest feeling of comfort. In reality, it is not actual comfort; it appears to be because we become used to our current state."[3]

If we learn to ignore our emotions, we become used to them and can subconsciously eat to comfort ourselves. The desensitizing tool causes us to subconsciously align with what others think and do, but this was never meant to be the case. Our emotions let us know whether or not we're being true to ourselves.

We must ask ourselves if we have subconsciously picked up some detrimental beliefs from others around us. Let me share an experience I had when our daughter with Down syndrome was five months old.

I went to a support group meeting for parents of children with Down syndrome (DS). The format was a panel discussion for parents (usually there was a speaker about a particular topic) to share their experiences. The first father shared about his son's hospitalization for corrective surgery. He spewed forth much bitterness with, "The doctors couldn't do this right, and the nurses didn't know what they were doing," etc. I left that meeting feeling discouraged and found myself acquiring bitter attitudes of my own. Subconsciously, I was adapting to these attitudes, which I didn't want to define me. This wasn't helpful. If anything, we needed a positive spirit encouraging us to see the good and to be hopeful. I decided not to return to those meetings unless there was a planned format with a speaker.

This is where sensitizing yourself comes in. A simple definition of *sensitize* is: "to make someone more aware of something."[4] My question to you is, "Are you aware of the attitudes you may be picking up from others around you?" Think about it. Do you have friends in the same situation as you are? Do you continue bad eating habits because everyone else is doing it? They're not going to care, so why do you need to? Have you desensitized yourself by rationalization, or could you now sensitize yourself to how you would like to be?

On page 12 in your journal, make a list of ways you have lulled yourself into being desensitized.

After you've done that, make another list of what you want for yourself. Are there people you can learn from? What about their attitudes and food choices? As you write them out, the ideas should flow. If not, get help from a trusted friend.

As you're now more aware of your desired outcome, please be more specific about what you would like. Is it more energy? To be healthier? To have your clothes fit better or not wonder how you look in them? To be more confident? To be happier and more at peace with yourself? Make your list now on page 13.

Now that you've done this, you must align your actions with your desired outcomes. This will take time to retrain your thinking and make decisions based on your new motivations as a first thought, not after-the-fact regret. Your future starts now, and you create it by the choices you make now. You have the ability to see a situation from both the negative and positive viewpoint. Example: "I want that piece of cake now, but I will regret it later" (negative), or "I can forgo that piece of cake, and I know I will feel good about the decision I made" (positive). Same situation—the cake—but how you respond determines the outcome. Your choices, however small or large, add up to create your reality and who you become. What do you want your destiny to look like?

Your future starts now, and you create it by the choices you make now.

In the next chapter, we will talk about our points of pain, including how we see and value ourselves. We need to learn to change our self-defeating thoughts and behaviors and to redefine empowering ourselves to take proactive steps. We are worth it, and we deserve better than how we've been treating ourselves. Keep reading!

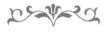

THE PROCESS

Chapter 5:
What Are My Pain Points? How Do They Affect My Self Concept?

"Today you are You, that is truer than true.
There is no one alive who is Youer than You."—Dr. Seuss

Pain—we all experience pain at different times in our lives, and we have different ways of dealing with it. For emotional pain, we can turn to alcohol, drugs, excessive work, video games, shopping, TV, or anything that's available to numb our feelings, including food. Food is readily available, and we have to eat. It's sometimes hard to detect when overeating is out of control. Deep down inside, we know when it has become a problem.

Sources of Pain

Physical Sources of Pain

There are several physical sources of pain that can cause you to want to eat. You have a bad night of sleep, and you're tired. Without even realizing it, you mindlessly eat to have more energy. You're aching all over for whatever reason (sleeping the wrong way, food allergies, coming down with a cold or the flu or having an autoimmune disease), and you use food unconsciously to make yourself feel better, but of course, it doesn't. You have no energy, and eating is your way to try to refuel yourself; in responding to your feelings, you don't make healthy choices.

Emotional Sources of Pain

Do you eat mindlessly? At times we eat to soothe our emotions because it has become a habit. If you think about it, you might discover you're bored or lonely. In AA, there's an acronym for triggers to drink: SALT—Sad, Angry, Lonely, Tired. If we check ourselves before starting to feed our emotional hunger, the appropriate accommodations can be made.

Other sources trigger emotional pain. Have you had conflict with a friend or a loved one and resorted to food? You've experienced losing a job, being violated in some way, feeling disrespected or rejected, feeling controlled, facing disappointments, and you eat for comfort. You can probably think of other areas I haven't mentioned.

As Joelle Casteix indicates in *The Power of Responsibility*, "We use food as an emotional crutch to avoid dealing with our pain and to 'bury our problems.' In the process it overtakes us and we lose what we want out of life."[1]

Many times, we use food as a "symbolic substitute." It becomes our best friend and takes the place of what we actually want and can't get. We look for a love connection, intimacy, or to feel good in the world, but somehow that seems to escape us. In the moment, we comfort ourselves with food to substitute for what we want but haven't been able to achieve.

Food is everywhere, and when you eat, you feel good; the pleasure centers in your brain are activated. Food becomes your faithful friend and a short-term solution, which can lead to addiction and become a cycle. Instead of having a symbolic substitute for what you desire, go after the real reward—connection, friendship, love, a meaningful job, or whatever it is that you want in your life.

Think of what's missing in your life. What are some possible ways of achieving it? Example: If you're lonely, where can you go to make friends? What about going to a meetup group (http://www.meetup.com) to find others with the same interests as you have, taking a class of interest or hobby, welcoming a new neighbor, involving yourself at church if you go, or volunteering? Go to page 14 in your journal to record your thoughts and possible action steps.

Other areas of pain can come from childhood issues of abuse or abandonment, being compared to a sibling, or receiving messages of "I'm not good enough" or "I have to be perfect to matter" or "I don't deserve better." If parents are unavailable for whatever reason, the child can internalize feelings of unworthiness. Oftentimes, we have core beliefs we're not even aware of.

Core Beliefs and Their Effect on Your Pain

When we have negative core beliefs about ourselves, it can wreak havoc in many areas of our lives—how we treat ourselves, our relationships with others, and decisions we make. We see people in toxic relationships, either as the recipient or as the one being toxic. What about people who let life circumstances get them down? Conversely, people who like themselves are happy, have good relationships, and are contributing members of society.

If we apply this to our weight struggles, we can see that when we care about ourselves, we do what's right for us; when we're struggling, it shows in our eating.

You may wonder what "how I see myself" has to do with your weight—number of calories eaten minus the number of calories expended equals weight loss or weight gain. It's as simple as that—a numbers game. While that may be true, that's not the whole story.

Your self-perception has everything to do with your weight. It plays a huge role in how you live your life, whether to boost your confidence or to sabotage it. This can be circular in nature. When we do something that sabotages our self-confidence, we feel down and continue to sabotage ourselves, not caring and not

Your self-perception has everything to do with your weight.

believing we deserve better. When we feel good about ourselves, we make choices that are in line with who we want to be and the expectations we have for ourselves. Our self-perception drives our behaviors to be congruent with what we believe we deserve out of life.

The Schema

When I was in graduate school, I learned about the term *schema. Merriam-Webster's Dictionary* defines it as, "a mental codification of experience that includes a particular organized way of perceiving cognitively and responding to a complex situation or set of stimuli."[2] In other words, your schema takes in whatever negative or positive thoughts you tell yourself. There's *no filter* to the schema. It believes what you tell it, whether it's true or false. If you tell yourself something that's *not* true, your schema takes it in as fact, does not question it in any way, and believes it. This shapes how you see and feel about yourself.

Let me share an example from my childhood. I remember standing in front of my mirror when I was about 9 or 10 years old (I can still see it as clearly as if it were yesterday). I don't know why I did this (maybe because I was chubby back in the day), but I looked at myself in the mirror and said, "You're ugly." I did this on many occasions until I began to believe it, and it didn't feel very good at all. To cheer myself up, I changed my mantra to "You're okay looking." Over time, I began to believe that, and it felt better. I began to accept my looks and who I was. Years later, I reframed it further with something like, "I'll never be Miss America, but I can be attractive in my own way." Then I took pride in my appearance and felt better about myself even more.

What is it about appearance anyway? We did nothing to deserve or earn it, so why do we let it define us? What about our wonderful qualities that make us who we are (fun loving, caring, smart, tenacious, organized, detail-oriented, etc.)? Our strengths and personality make us who we are, and that's what we need to embrace—all the good qualities we have, so it resonates and becomes our authentic selves.

Your schema believes you—what you tell yourself is *so important*! From our schema, come our thoughts, feelings, and actions. Our thoughts are very powerful and can evoke emotion at the drop of a hat. When our son went to Iraq serving in the United States Army, I was a basket case for a while. Whenever I thought of the "black car" coming to bring news of his death, I began to cry. It was automatic. No holding back the tears. After a few weeks of this unproductive use of my time and emotions, I tried something else. Did I trust myself enough to get through the tragedy of his death, if it did happen? Yes, it would be sad, very sad, more than sad, but I knew with a good support system, I would make it. With that realization, I no longer had to worry about the "black car." I would be okay, and it freed me to not be imprisoned by my fears.

Let's take this one step further. Our belief systems drive our thoughts, which drive our feelings, which drive our actions. Take, for instance, a man who believes all women are cheaters. He comes home from a long business trip and finds his wife/girlfriend not there. He immediately thinks she's out cheating on him. He fumes, and when she comes home, he yells and throws her around. Had she done anything to make him mad? No. It was his belief that triggered his thoughts, emotions, and behaviors.

Now let's look at another man who has the belief system that women can be trusted. He comes home from his long business trip, and she is not there. He begins to unpack his suitcase, realizing she may be at the grocery store, running errands, or out with friends. When she comes home, he stops his unpacking and greets her with a kiss and a hug, tells her how much he missed her, and that he's glad to see her. Same scenario, but two different belief systems, which affect thoughts, emotions, and behaviors.

Why is this important? What we believe about ourselves determines our thoughts, feelings, and actions, and this will affect our actions around food. We can be triggered into overeating, if we subconsciously don't feel good about ourselves or struggle with some unresolved issue. Feeling down, we turn to food. Self-sabotaging behaviors are common because our feelings drive our actions, and we eat to feel better, but, of course, we don't. This can set up a self-fulfilling prophecy, and we shrink in despair.

Effect of Your Background

Our self-image plays a vital role in our successes or failures in life. It entails how we think and feel about who we are and how we perceive ourselves to be in this world. As Jim Thomson shares in his book, *The Formula for Christian Self Esteem,* our self-image is formed by the value others place on us while growing up, and it's formed over time. If parents spend time with their children and value their strengths and who they are as little people, they will develop a good self-image. If, on the other hand, they are neglected or abused in any way, they can develop a poor self-image and react negatively in adverse circumstances. This continues into adolescence and the adult years.[3]

Thomson uses the analogy of a blank slate, which we come into this world with and which is written upon over time. We take in all the ways we're valued or devalued and form our self-perception from the way people treat us. The important relationships in our lives (family) have the most impact, but others contribute to it as well. No one incident defines us completely, and we can determine how it impacts us by our interpretation of the incident. It's not what happens to us,

It's not what happens to us, but what we tell ourselves about the event that determines our feelings and actions.

but what we tell ourselves about the event that determines our feelings and actions.

Your Parents' Upbringing Can Affect Your Sense of Self

As an adult now, it's important to separate your perception from childhood to seeing your parents' background and its impact on you. Others' behaviors are more about them than about you, although it's easy to internalize as such.

Do you know what it was like for your parents as they were growing up? Were they loved and nurtured, or was their home dysfunctional with domestic violence, a lot of conflict, drinking or drugs, and physical and/or verbal abuse? Were they left to themselves and neglected of emotional connection, or were they affirmed and encouraged in their endeavors?

If a mother or father, as a child, had always been told they weren't good enough, had to perform to be accepted, were abused, etc., and they passed down their legacy, this in no way implies the child is incompetent or unlovable. It's simply what they're bringing to the table, but the child internalizes the message personally.

This does not excuse our parents' behaviors toward us. Sometimes, it helps to see it more objectively and to help us know that their behavior toward us isn't about who we are; it's about them continuing to pass down their legacy from what they knew.

We have to take responsibility for how we're going to live, so our past doesn't bleed into our future.

However, this in no way gives us an excuse to bury our

sorrows in food. We have to take responsibility for how we're going to live, so our past doesn't bleed into our future.

Childhood Circumstances

Our parents, family, friends, and acquaintances influence who we become as we grow up. Circumstances can as well. They can be simple things, such as small upsets, but could have a lasting impact. Let me give you a few examples.

Karen is busy in the kitchen, trying to coordinate getting dinner together on time, and she doesn't acknowledge her toddler's plea for attention. The toddler doesn't know how to communicate her hurt, and she internalizes not feeling worthy of her mother's attention, not realizing it has nothing to do with her worth.

Joseph has abandoned the family. His small daughter, Suzie, doesn't have the vocabulary to express her feelings of how scared and alone she feels. At two, all Suzie knows is that "Daddy left." She can carry these feelings of abandonment, of not being lovable, and that something is wrong with her, into adulthood. It becomes a part of who she is, without being aware of it. She doesn't know what life is like any other way. This empty feeling causes her to turn to food.

Imagine Donna winning first place in a competition and her mother questions if she really did. Not being believed she could actually win a competition causes her to seek validation from those who believe she is capable, and perfectionism sets in. As an adult, she resorts to the comfort of food for validation without even realizing it.

Perhaps from your childhood, you were given messages that you didn't matter, that you weren't good enough, that you had to perform to a certain standard to be accepted, that you were worthless and unlovable. This is so *not* true, but, as a child, this became engrained into your psyche. You don't know any other way to think or feel. This is who you are. You take all these circumstances with you into adulthood.

You may have had significant trauma in your life, grew up in a dysfunctional home, or had losses that have yet to be mourned. This could entail "disenfranchised losses" that might include a lot of moving, loss of a job, having a wayward child, unfulfilled expectations, loss of the marriage you had hoped for through divorce, etc. Unresolved trauma can also impact who you become.

If you've had experiences as mentioned above, consider seeing a counselor who can help you work through many of these issues that may be keeping you stuck. Trust me; there *is* a better way to live.

Negative and Positive Self-Talk

People who feel good about who they are talk to themselves differently than those who don't like themselves. We have an inner dialogue, which can be positive or negative. It's the chatter that goes on in our minds without our realizing it.

If we're too hard on ourselves, we tend to be self-critical with thoughts, such as, "I should have done better," or "How could I be so dumb?" When we engage in negative self talk, it degrades the very fiber of our sense of self. If we can be more compassionate toward ourselves with statements, such as, "It was a hard

When we engage in negative self-talk, it degrades the very fiber of our sense of self.

test," or "I could have studied more," we will keep our self-image intact.

If you look at these responses, the negative self-talk comes from focusing on internal forces of "not being good enough" or feeling incompetent and unworthy. This causes a loss in motivation and in feeling happiness in knowing you're worthwhile. You can become a perfectionist to avoid showing you're flawed.

Positive self-talk comes from seeing external circumstances coming into play as opposed to internal flaws of character. You don't take it personally. This way, you're able to improve future performance without condemning yourself; you can learn from your mistakes and move on. When you feel good about who you are, you can be productive and move forward with your goals.

Do any of the following concepts resonate with you? These can result in negative core beliefs.

- I only had conditional love, if I had any love at all.
- I raised myself and was neglected.
- I was rejected by those I cared about.
- I was not listened to by the important people in my life.
- I had unrealistic expectations placed on me (too high or too low).
- I was compared to others in a negative light.
- I was used and abused.

On a positive note,

- I felt accepted, respected, and loved.
- I felt connected and bonded with loved ones.
- I was listened to.
- I had my wants and needs met.
- I saw myself as a unique individual.
- I knew I made good decisions.
- I grew up being healthy and in good shape.
- I am responsible and take responsibility for my actions.
- I can forgive myself and learn from my mistakes.
- I have a sense of purpose in life.

Healing the Pain

We are self-medicating when we use food to numb our feelings. We need to go back to the feelings we are suppressing to find healing. With food, we want momentary relief from being bored, tired, sad, angry, etc. We must deal with these feelings instead of resorting to food.

Forgiveness

Before we can do any kind of healing when we have been hurt by others, it's necessary to forgive those who have hurt us. This isn't to say that whatever they did to us was alright; whatever it was, we didn't deserve it. For our own sake, we need to forgive to break the negative bond we have with that person. We do it for us. It has been said that not forgiving and holding a grudge is like drinking poison and waiting for someone else to die.

What are the components of forgiveness?

- It's a choice we consciously make; it's not a feeling.
- We must let go of feeling sorry for ourselves.
- We must face the wrong that was done to us.
- We must recognize the emotions we're feeling.
- We must choose to not hold it against them.
- We must release them.
- If we don't forgive, we will continue to be imprisoned by our resentments, bitterness, and anger.
- Because forgiveness can be a process, we must forgive on a daily basis, if needed. This sets us free!

Before moving on, think about those in your life you need to forgive. If you need a place to write this down, go to page 15 in your journal. There you can walk through the steps listed above.

Beginning the Healing

Now that you've dealt with unfinished business, it's time to internalize the concepts to see yourself in a new way, to empower yourself to no longer be a victim to the lure of food, but rather to take back your life!

On page 16 in your journal, list what you like about yourself. What are your strengths? What do others like about you? What do they see as your strengths?

Have these messages been lost in the negative self-chatter that goes on in your head? Do you stop to challenge them? Or do they reign supreme? List the negative thoughts that swirl around in your head. Don't keep reading until you've done this. Seriously. List them on page 16 in your journal. We will develop these further in Chapter 6.

I want you to play devil's advocate. You must challenge your negative self-talk, or it will go into your schema as true. Are these thoughts really true? What if you said, "I'm fat; nobody's going to want me." You don't know that. We call that "predicting the future" or "fortune telling." Probably many people out there share common interests with you and would love your sense of humor or other strengths. If you do weigh more than you should, you can do something about it, and this book is intended to help you do that.

You must challenge your negative self-talk, or it will go into your schema as true.

Here's another example: What if you said, "I've always been fat, and I'll never be trim." That is "all-or-nothing" thinking. You know that on True/False questions on a test, if the words *always* or *never* are in the statement, the answer is usually **false**. Just because you've been overweight all your life doesn't mean you have to stay that way. Maybe it was modeled behavior, or you came from an environment with all the wrong foods, and you had no choice because the food was provided by the adults in your life. You have choices now. Will making the change in eating habits be difficult? Probably. Can you do it? Absolutely! You have to want to change and commit to making it happen. You have to want the change more than you want the *momentary* pleasures of indulgence. Challenge those negative thoughts, and claim a new day for yourself. You can do this!

You can't change your negative beliefs that are driving your behaviors if you don't acknowledge them. If you don't see yourself as being worthy, you won't believe you deserve better. You may think, *Ho hum, this is my lot in life,* and you continue with self-sabotaging behaviors. You want more out of life, but you don't think you deserve it, so you don't go after it. It's time for that way of thinking to end. Once and for all!

The next chapter will lay the groundwork for resetting or tapping into your core sense of self. Here you will find your strength to deal with temptations and sabotaging behaviors, both your own and from others. You will jump over the obstacles that have and will continue to pose a challenge in your weight-loss journey. Please keep reading ...

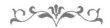

Chapter 6:
Where Does My Change Begin?

"Do not let the hero in your soul perish in lonely frustration for the life you deserved and have never been able to reach. The world you desire can be won. It exists... it is real... it is possible. It's yours."—Ayn Rand, *Atlas Shrugged*

Let this quote resonate with you. The life you want is attainable. You have to want it more than anything; when you do, you're on your way to obtain what you have previously been unable to attain and maintain.

In the last chapter, we learned how our self-concept is important to our weight-loss efforts. It drives our emotions and behaviors. It's fundamental to the integrity of the very fiber of our being. It affects the choices we make and who we become.

When you feel good about yourself, you make choices that are congruent with who you perceive yourself to be. If you have self-worth and believe you deserve that job, that promotion, that education, that whatever-it-may-be, you go after it, whatever it takes. You may not get it, but that doesn't stop you from the next opportunity. You spring into action, taking proactive initiative to search for and pursue the next thing that will propel you forward with your goals for your life. You have goals; you believe you're worth it and deserve to have a good life. You go after it, to claim what is rightfully yours.

You must begin the process of creating a positive sense of self that allows you to pursue your weight-loss goals with success. It won't happen overnight, but you can do this. You're probably not even aware of the negative thoughts that run rampant in your head.

Dealing with the Effect of Your Childhood and Your Core Beliefs

On page 18 in your journal, think about how you grew up. What messages did you internalize? Did you feel that what you did was never "good enough"? Or that you had to be perfect? Or that you were "invisible"? The list of core beliefs in childhood in Chapter 5 may spur your thinking. Think about any messages from your childhood that might sabotage your weight-loss and weight-management efforts. Challenge them and create your own affirmations about who you are and who you want to become.

Self-Talk

Negative Self-Talk

We *all* have negative thoughts we experience daily. On a recent Dr. Phil Show, he asked the audience how many people have negative thoughts on a daily basis to please raise their hands. Not only did the entire audience raise their hands, but Dr. Phil raised BOTH hands! We all do it. The key point is to challenge those thoughts, reframe them, and not let them take control and residence in our lives.

On page 20 in your journal, list your negative thoughts you need to challenge. Don't let them have power over you! Are they true or not true? I think you will find they're not true. If you believe they are, ask a trusted friend to validate or negate them. When you have your list, take each negative thought, challenge it, and reframe it with a positive way of seeing yourself.

Example: I think others are critical of me. Challenge: You don't know that they are, and what if they are? Reframe: I know I have good qualities, and I like being me. If the reframe is uncomfortable, you have some work to do.

Keep a running log of your thoughts, both positive and negative. Ask yourself if these thoughts make you feel better or worse about yourself. Of those that make you feel worse, find a different way to think, such as, "I can learn from my mistakes," or "I am good at _____," or "I can start afresh," etc. We'll talk more about this in Chapter 7 on cognitive distortions. Keep up the good work on your positive self-talk! That's the fuel that will drive your engine to success.

Are you busy thinking and focusing on your negative thoughts about yourself, your weaknesses, and where you fall short? Have you taken time to consider your good qualities and given voice to them? You've just *listed* your negative thoughts, *challenged*, and *reframed* them, so you can raise your awareness of how much you fall into this pattern. Don't let your negative thoughts crowd out your positive ones. When you're stuck in these negative thought processes, it prevents you from feeling good about who you are and keeps you from pursuing your dreams and goals.

"If you're only looking at the past and focusing on the negative, that's where your brain will take you," according to Joelle Casteix in her book, *The Power of Responsibility*. She goes on to say, "And where you are going is totally in your control."[1] We don't need to stay mired down by our past; we can choose a new trajectory for our lives.

Our self-talk affects how we see things in life. Look at the following picture. What do you see? Do you see the old hag or the beautiful woman? We can look on the negative side of life and see "the old hag" or we go through life with a more positive lens and see "the beautiful woman." Which do you choose?

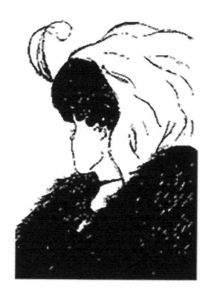

Positive Self-Talk

Now it's time to shift your focus to your strengths and positive qualities. When you see yourself more favorably, you will feel more empowered to pursue your dreams and goals and claim the right to be more fit, healthier, and happier.

Finding Your Strengths and Positive Qualities

In your journal on page 22, make a list of your strengths and positive qualities. You may say, "I don't have any" or "I don't know of any." We all have something that makes us unique and special. Are you a caring parent or kind to animals? What are your talents? Are you good at art or have an ear for music?

What about your innate characteristics? Are you detailed-oriented, analytical, organized? Maybe you're more of a big-picture thinker, have lots of ideas and possibilities. You get the idea. If you need help with this assignment, ask some friends or family who know you to help.

In my counseling practice, I had a client who was struggling with this. He had a social get-together with his friends, and they came up with 47 strengths he had, some of which he never would have thought of or seen on his own. His friends were objective and saw qualities he had quashed or never allowed himself to embrace. If you don't have friends close by, send them an email, google "List of Strengths," or check out http://www.viacharacter.org for character strengths.

As Dr. Marilyn J. Sorensen describes in her book, *Breaking the Chain of Low Self-Esteem*, keep a record of these strengths and character qualities nearby so you can review them three to five times a day. Using 3 x 5 cards, a journal, or a notebook will help. Decide on something that is user-friendly, so you will do this. Carry it with you to have easy access throughout the day. It's important to verbally go over your strengths, preferably in front of a mirror.[2] (There's something about the mirror that reinforces belief. Remember my mirror story?) If you do that, you will begin to believe these truths about yourself. Remember the schema? You have to feed these positive truths into your schema, so eventually you will embrace them as who you are.

You should consider going through the process of reviewing your strengths for six months or as long as it takes. Let me give you an example while growing up. Although I had lost weight when I was 11, some of the pounds gradually returned in my teens. After losing those pounds again and keeping them off, I saw my reflection in the mirror as a trim young lady, but it didn't register emotionally with me. After about three years, it finally hit me, "I'm not fat!" I ran to my brother in amazement and said, "I'm not fat!" He looked at me as if I had lost my mind and said, "Of course, you're not!" He probably wondered what in the world I was thinking! I could see it in the mirror intellectually, but emotionally I had not yet internalized it until that moment.

I could see it in the mirror intellectually, but emotionally I had not yet internalized it until that moment.

This process for you to make a mind shift will take some time, hopefully not three years. That's why using your cards or your journal three to five times a day, preferably in front of a mirror, will facilitate this transformation. Instead of focusing on the negative all the time, it's important to give voice to your strengths while recognizing areas you can improve. When you lose your weight, you can use this same process to internalize your new self-image of being slim and trim.

Isn't it time you feasted at the banquet of life, claiming all the blessings that are out there for you? You can grab onto a better life. Don't let your weight issues hold you back. It's time!

Affirmations

While you're doing this, don't forget to include affirmations, which are positive statements of empowerment. As Hal Elrod describes in his book, *The Miracle Morning*, you want them to reflect what you want and why you want it.[3] They should be short, direct, and in the present tense or present progressive tense (I am becoming _____). You should ask yourself if you're committed to becoming and doing what it will take to change your life. Here are some sample statements:

- I will find ways to be successful.

- I am strong.

- I desire to and I will lose weight.

- I desire to be healthy with more energy, and I will achieve it.

It's time to make some of your own. Turn to page 24 in your journal. List what it is you desire for your life, whether it refers to your weight goals, marriage and family goals, business goals, etc. Think about your emotions behind the affirmations. What will you stand to gain? What will you lose if you don't accomplish your goals? Make sure these goals have emotional impact in the new trajectory you desire for your life. Will you take ownership of these affirmations every

Change comes through our emotions, not our intellect...

time you review them? Change comes through our emotions, not our intellect; it's important to be emotionally invested in them.

"Self-Talk" Buddy

Sometimes, we have a hard time believing we have worth. A trusted friend can help. Your "self talk" buddy will read or say your affirmations back to you. This can be done in person, on the phone with FaceTime, or by Skyping. This helps to reinforce what you might not dare to believe on your own. Belief is strengthened by the support of others. You can return the favor in an area that is important to your friend.

Reshaping Your Mindset

In Jerry Minchinton's book, *Maximum Self-Esteem*, he describes how self-perception affects feelings and behaviors. As you begin to reshape your mindset and core beliefs about yourself, you will appreciate your value as a human being, accept yourself more fully, become comfortable in your own skin, and value your uniqueness and contribution to the world, however big or small that may be.[4]

You respect yourself and know that you matter, to yourself and to others. You appreciate your personal worth. You feel good about who you are, coming from the inside out, without needing others to validate you. You like you for you, says Minchinton, regardless of external compliments.

When you feel good about who you are, you find it is easier to control your emotions. For the most part, you're free from core emotions of guilt, fear, sadness, and anger. Yes, at times, they pop up, but they don't define your daily life. If you're not there yet, keep working on changing your core beliefs about your value and worth. You *will* get there, and you *will* be amazed at how much better you feel and act! Out of this comes your happiness, simply because you like who you have now become.

When you have a positive image of yourself, you're not afraid to try something new because of fear of failing. If you fail, you learn from it, and you don't limit yourself by that failure. You set goals, and you believe you can attain them. Minchinton states that when you do this, you embrace your accomplishments. This has now become congruent with your sense of self.

If we act as though we deserve to be treated with disrespect, others will treat us that way. If we believe we have worth, we carry ourselves in such a way with confidence that commands respect. It doesn't take a rocket scientist to spot someone who feels good about himself by the very way he carries himself, looks you in the eye, and shakes your hand.

These chapters on how we see and treat ourselves and how we can make the change happen are important because they provide the basis for making change. We have to believe our worth and that we deserve better. We cannot improve our lives outwardly if inwardly we don't believe we deserve the result of making these changes.

> *We cannot improve our lives outwardly if ... we don't believe we deserve the result of making these changes.*

In summary, using the information in this chapter, you will:

- Make a list of limiting beliefs.
- Challenge and reframe negative thoughts.

- Make a list of strengths, character qualities, and positive behaviors.

- Make a list of positive affirmations of your value and actions you will take.

- Get a "self-talk" buddy.

- Review strengths and affirmations every day three to five times in front of a mirror.

In the next chapter on cognitive distortions, we will look at challenging our thought processes in more detail, which will help us to defeat our own worst enemy lurking within us—our thoughts.

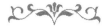

Chapter 7: "Stinkin' Thinkin'" (Cognitive Distortions)

"Change your thoughts and you change your world."
—Norman Vincent Peale

"Oops! I blew it!" We all have times when we give in to temptation and later wish we hadn't. How will you respond to this minor lapse in judgment? Will you recognize it as such and move on? Will you blow it out of proportion and beat yourself up with never-ending self-deprecation? Will you be disgusted with yourself and turn to food for comfort, making the problem worse?

Mistakes happen. One event will not do you in; what you tell yourself about what just happened will. For instance, you say things like, "I'm such a loser," or "I'm always going to be this way," or "I'm disgusted with myself," or "This is terrible," or "Others will see me as a fat pig," and on and on you go. Instead, try looking at it a little differently by being kind to yourself with the realization that tomorrow is another day (or if you binged in the morning, you can end the binge now). Turn your negative thoughts into positive ones. "Yes, I made a mistake. It doesn't have to define me. I can get back into healthy eating patterns and move forward in reaching the outcome I desire."

Think about it this way. If you overspend one day, will you be bankrupt the next day? No, but if you continue to overspend, you will head for financial disaster and possible bankruptcy. Bankruptcy doesn't happen overnight. It comes with a long history of not paying your bills (caveat, sometimes there are unforeseen circumstances, such as a large medical bill above and beyond insurance coverage) and continuing to rack up credit card debt. It's easy to get into the habit of "I want what I want when I want it" and suffer the consequences of short-term gratification.

The same is true with overeating. One day of overeating won't make you fat; it's the day-after-day of overeating or eating the wrong foods that will. Conversely, if you're reading this and you need to lose weight, one good day won't make it happen, but day-after-day of healthy eating habits will reap the rewards you're looking for.

How is it possible to put all those good days into practice? If you think of setting up an accountability system for yourself, use a calendar to mark off the days you've been successful in maintaining control of your eating. Every day you put an X down, you're setting up a chain of good behaviors and accountability. This is called chaining. It has been said that when Jerry Seinfeld was an unknown, he wrote a joke a day, at least one joke. When he had, he marked the day on the calendar with an X as succeeding for that day. Late at night if he had not written a joke, he made sure that he did so he could mark it off. He didn't want to break the chain. We know of Jerry's success; it started out simply, consistently writing one joke at a time, building up over time to where it became as natural as breathing.

You can have success, one small step at a time. If you stumble, catch yourself before you spiral out of control. This is the time to check your self-talk. You cannot allow yourself to go down that path. It's time to break negative self-fulfilling behaviors. Instead of victimizing yourself, take a

If you stumble, catch yourself before you spiral out of control.

step toward reframing all those cognitive distortions with right thinking. Cognitive distortions are simply "stinkin' thinkin'," to coin a phrase from grad school. They're the thoughts that are distorted and get us into trouble.

Dr. David Burns, in his book, *The Feeling Good Handbook: The New Mood Therapy,* describes 10 of the most common distortions. Let's look at some of them:[1]

"All-or-nothing thinking." People who fall into this category tend to think in black and white. There's no room for other possibilities, and there are no "gray" areas. These people tend to be rigid and cause stress by their very rigid nature. We have to think about the possibility of other ways to act. "I made a mistake; I'm a total failure." No, mistakes happen, and we can pick ourselves up and move on. Mistakes don't make us failures. We all make mistakes; it's how we react to those mistakes that define who we are and who we become. We can wallow in our self-pity and verbally abuse ourselves for that one mistake, or we can learn from it, move on, and grow from it to become stronger, more well-balanced people.

"Overgeneralization." This happens when we make a mistake and globalize it to be a never-ending pattern. "I didn't get the job, as usual." "Well, what else do you expect from me," might be your thought process. Instead of seeing your mistake as a never-ending pattern, you can look at it as one event in time. Maybe it wasn't the job for you, or there could be a better job out there. Sometimes we think we cannot break out of these patterns, which we think define us. We can begin new ways of thinking that will serve us well in the future as we recognize these thought patterns that get in our way.

"Fortune-telling" or "predicting the future." We are predicting the future when we say, "I made a mistake. I will always make these same mistakes." We don't know that. Will our expectations of failing become a self-fulfilling prophecy? Did you also pick up on the other two cognitive distortions previously mentioned? The words *always* and *never* are polarizing words, a sign of black-and-white or all-or-nothing thinking. There's also overgeneralization with the never-ending pattern of thinking.

"Jumping to conclusions." Carly is expected to attend an upcoming social event. She wants to see everyone and connect socially, but she's afraid of her response to all the tempting food. She hasn't had success with willpower in the past. Subconsciously, she tells herself, "I know I'm going to cave and sample too much of everything." Does she really know that?

Can you relate to Carly? You may have done the same thing in the past without a plan, and you may also have allowed yourself to do so by rationalizing. Remember what rationalizing does. It gives us permission to do something we know we shouldn't by giving a reason why it is okay to do so (rational lies!). Don't! If you really want to have a good time without regrets, why not come up with a game plan of how to navigate the evening with some kind of accountability built in? You may decide to have fruits and vegetables and allow yourself one treat within reason (or not). You can have the person you go with help you with accountability (see Chapter 12), or if you're going alone, you may decide to tell a friend your plan and report back. There's nothing like accountability to keep us on the straight-and-narrow.

"Discounting the positive." Jason discounts his positive behaviors and focuses on the negative ones. He has a good week of self-control and loses a few pounds but then succumbs to temptation. That's all he can think about, that he messed up, that he's lousy at losing weight, and what a failure he is for giving in to temptation. He gives no thought or credit for the success he had earlier in the week. If he shifted his thinking to realize he has been successful this week with a minor slip-up, he can get back on track instead of falling into a pit of despair.

"Mental filter." It's easy to pick out one negative detail that colors our thinking for the rest of the day, like putting on sunglasses when there's no need to. Think of a glass of water being darkened by a single drop of food coloring. If we eat a little too much at breakfast, does it affect our eating the rest of the day because we've already blown it? It doesn't have to! Only if we let it.

Here are some other cognitive distortions. "Catastrophizing" is when the problem is made out to be much worse than it is ("the sky is falling"), and "minimizing" keeps us from recognizing the full impact of our wrong choices. "Emotional reasoning" comes into play when we say something such as, "I feel like a fat pig." This assumes negative feelings reflect reality rather than having made a mistake. "Labeling" is attributing behaviors to a person's character. "I'm a failure." A mistake doesn't define us as failures; it's just a mistake. "Personalization" is taking responsibility for something bad happening, even though it's not about us at all.

"Should statements" get many of us into trouble just about every day. We should do this; we should do that; if only I had done _____; I shouldn't have done that. Is this the voice that runs rampant in our heads? Are we being too hard on ourselves? Are our expectations too high? Others aren't putting those expectations on us; we are. We need to stop it! Yes, it's important to have high standards, if that is what we value, but at what cost to our emotional health when we don't come through for ourselves?

The gap between our expectations and reality produces anger. If we're not living up to the expectations we place on ourselves, we become angry and disappointed. We take it out on ourselves in self-hatred, disgust, guilt, and shame. This is no way to live. Aren't you tired of being upset with yourself every time you fall short of your expectations? Where is your resiliency to bounce back? When will you show up for yourself? If an adult were verbally abusing your child, you would step in to protect them. When will you step in to protect yourself from yourself? When will you show up for you? If you don't, who will?

The gap between our expectations and reality produces anger.

Is there a tendency toward perfectionism? Are you falling short of your own ideals? Perfection doesn't exist because we all make mistakes. That's what makes us human and relatable to others. Is there a better way to think about your own ideals? You want to have high standards (if you do), but when you mess up and fall short of your own "shoulds," isn't it time to be kind to yourself with, "Yes, I messed up; I'm not perfect. I wanted to do _____, but I didn't. I'll figure out a way to do better next time." If you can ease up on yourself, you will be more relaxed and able to enjoy the process more on the way to a new you. Remember: it's a process, and there will be ups and downs in the journey, but you will get there if you don't jump ship.

Before moving on, go to page 26 in your journal to identify some of your cognitive distortions. Which ones plague you? How can you challenge and reframe them? This is where the rubber meets the road. Your self-talk will define you—whether you become a victim or the victor!

Your self-talk will define you—whether you become a victim or the victor!

In the next chapter, we will learn how to internalize a new body image and self-image that match how we want to conduct our lives with confidence and freedom. Keep reading to find out how to do that.

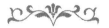

Chapter 8:
Creating My New Identity

"Courage is looking FEAR in the eye and saying,
'Get out of my way; I've got things to do.'"
—Unknown

Consider creating a new identity for yourself where you have a body image and self-image that match, where you feel good about yourself and your body shows it. You feel vibrant and alive and ready to conquer whatever the day holds in front of you. You're ready and eager! What would that mean for you to create that kind of life? But you say, "That's not me; I could never be *that* person." Why not? Deep down inside, you are that person. You have allowed your weight to hold you back and not be the confident, happy person you know you can be. Isn't it time to allow the real you to shine forth?

It is possible to change. In order to do so, you must stop making excuses and begin to believe you're worth the hard work and the new life ahead.

The Problem of Resistance

In the field of psychology, we sometimes see people who aren't making much progress. We have to ask ourselves, "What is causing this person to remain stuck?" There are two concepts I'd like to share with you. They're called outcome resistance and process resistance.

Outcome Resistance

Outcome resistance is a term used when we're afraid to make new changes and what the "new life" will look like when those changes are made. Are you afraid to have more required of you? Joseph finds that it's easier to watch his family play Frisbee on the beach rather than getting involved, and others don't require more of him. Linda is afraid to lose the friends she loves to eat out with at all the restaurants that serve too much food. Somewhere along the way, you get a payoff for remaining overweight. You're afraid you will lose something—camaraderie with friends, maybe your relationship with your spouse (he/she could be threatened by your changing and miss the status quo), losing foods you love. You fear loss, so you stay stuck.

You fear loss, so you stay stuck.

On page 28 in your journal, think about what your payoffs are. You might not think you have any, but you do. If you need help, ask a friend or family member. When you see the reasons why you're stuck in your weight issues, that can be the "aha" you need. When you have that "aha" moment, you can start on a new path, to claim the life you desire that is rightfully yours!

Instead of focusing on what you will lose, focus on the benefits you will gain in making these changes. While you're at it, think of how your life will change positively when you conquer your fears of having a new outcome in your life. What will be different? Will you have more quality time with your children? Your spouse? Will your sex life improve? More energy for work? Make your list on page 28 of what new outcomes you hope for.

We have now figured out why we're resistant to making the change, and we want a better life for ourselves. It's time to look at the difficulties we may face in actually trying to make the change. Let's turn our focus to *process resistance.*

Process Resistance

Changing behavior is hard work! We're comfortable eating the foods we love with minimal exercise, if any at all; we don't want to give up our comfortable habits. When you begin a diet, you will need to plan new menus, change your shopping routines, learn to cook in healthier ways, and begin to exercise, if you're not already doing so. (Check with your doctor first.)

Part of process resistance also includes the fear of loss—loss of a comfortable lifestyle, giving up foods you love and a lifestyle that revolves around food. Instead of thinking of what you will lose, think of new ways of being around food and what you will gain by doing so.

When you begin your new way of eating, you will enjoy tasting the fresh flavor of foods you formerly shunned. Instead of avoiding social functions around food, you have found new ways to manage your eating habits in spite of triggers and self-sabotaging behavior (Chapters 9 and 10). You will be delighted to shop for a new wardrobe and feel good in your new look.

What if, instead of being overwhelmed by making these changes, you saw it as a challenge that would make you a winner on the other side? What if you visualized and delighted in the process of change, to become your best self? How motivating would that be! Isn't it time to put yourself first, including conquering your weight struggles, by committing and believing you can make these changes?

It is possible to change. In order to do so, you must stop making excuses and begin to believe you're worth the hard work and the new life ahead.

Mirror Neurons

You've heard the expression, "Fake it till you make it." It can work in your favor to see yourself in a new light. The brain has "mirror neurons" which bring about what is projected onto them, according to Dr. Nancy Irwin in her weblog, *Mirror, Mirror on the Brain.* We talked about the schema not knowing the difference between what's real and what's not. When you see a scary movie, your heart starts to beat faster, you may sweat, and you're scared. You know the danger is not real, but you react as if it were.[1]

You can use this process to "trick" your mind into achieving new goals. Dr. Irwin goes on to describe what happens with the "mirror neurons." If you imagine making that perfect free throw on the basketball court, your mirror neurons "hold" that image of making the free throw, so it actually believes you can do it. Brain scans confirm this activity, whether you're shooting free throws or just thinking about it.

If you set aside some time each day (preferably before bed so you can sleep on it and again in the morning), write out your "fantasy" (the dream you want to believe but don't at this point). This comes with acting in a way that's congruent with your goals. Dr. Irwin states that when you "fake it till you make it," you know these mirror neurons are working in your favor to change how you see yourself. Try it! You have nothing to lose and a new way of living to gain.

Creating a New Body Image

Where the mind goes, actions follow. This is played out in every area of our lives. It begins with believing you deserve and want this new healthy and energized version of yourself. If this is not where you are now, you have some work to do.

Where the mind goes, actions follow.

Did you know that healthier, leaner people have a conscious goal about their weight *and* an unconscious positive identity or self-image? You may have a conscious weight goal but an unconscious negative body image that can thwart your conscious goals.

What do I mean by that? You can desire to lose weight, but if you see yourself as being overweight and not envisioning the new you, it's easy to fall back into patterns that sustain the extra weight. Have you known people who have lost weight only to gain it all back (and then some)? If you maintain your overweight body image you had before losing weight, it's easy to subconsciously return to that same image.

If you maintain your overweight body image ... it's easy to subconsciously return to that same image.

Those who are healthier and leaner have a conscious goal of their weight and an unconscious identity/self-image where they think, feel, and act a certain way that keeps them consistently at their desired weight. When this new body image is internalized, it helps to sustain your new weight because you make decisions that will support maintaining your new slim self.

Our conscious mind is where we set out goals. Willpower and persistence are played out consciously and work in the short term. Our unconscious mind sends us back to our comfort zone and how we envision ourselves. It's important to visualize how we want to feel and act in our new body; if we don't, our unconscious mind takes over to what we're accustomed to, and we're right back to where we started, having gained the weight back.

Our unconscious mind sends us back to our comfort zone and how we envision ourselves.

How many people set a goal in the beginning of the new year to lose weight and exercise, but they later lose motivation and abandon their goals within a few weeks? Maybe you can relate. When we make New Year's resolutions, we choose our goals (consciously) but don't create a new body image we can visualize and believe we deserve (unconsciously). Is this why yo-yo dieting is so prevalent? We consciously lose the weight, but unconsciously, we haven't internalized this new image, and we gradually regain the weight to return to the old

We ... lose the weight, but ... we haven't internalized this new image, and we ... regain the weight to return to the old overweight image.

overweight image. *If you get nothing else out of this book, please understand and apply this concept!*

We must reset our self-image and our body image. Did you know that people who perceive themselves to be heavier actually gain weight? Interesting. This is where visualization is important. *Visualization* can be defined as "the formation of mental visual images, the act or process of interpreting in visual terms or of putting into visible form."[2] You have to see it in your mind's eye.

On page 30 in your journal, visualize what your new body will look like. What will you be wearing? What kind of energy will you have? Will you be confident, or will your posture betray you? Will there be a smile on your face and a look that says, "I can conquer the world"? Think about your new body image and how you will feel when you accomplish your goals.

This is what you will use when you get to The Plan stage. As you begin and continue on your journey, you will become more confident and free from all the time you spend thinking about food and your weight. Your body image and self-image will be aligned with who you want to be. Joelle Casteix says in *The Power of Responsibility*, "The only things that matter are who you are right now and the kind of person you decide to be from this moment onward."[3] You can become that person who wakes up ready to conquer the world!

In the meantime, let's look at our triggers that so readily entice us to give in to the short-term gratification of eating what we know we shouldn't. Can we figure out a way to find better coping skills with temptations? Please keep reading ...

Chapter 9:
Watch Your Triggers!

"Self-knowledge is better than self-control any day," Raquel said firmly. "And I know myself well enough to know how I act around cookies."—Claudia Gray, *Evernight*

Triggers are everywhere. You walk down the street past a bakery, and the aroma lures you in. You see the decadent food others are having at a restaurant, and you think, "I want that, too!" A trigger is something that begins a chain reaction. It can be caused by feeling emotional pain or seeing or smelling the lure of easy comfort food readily available. It's the "cocking of the gun" before giving in and pulling the trigger. Nothing happens if you don't pull the trigger; if you allow it to overtake you, the resulting damage and devastation ensue. The damage results in gaining a few pounds, but the real damage comes in the price you pay in self-hatred, self-deprecation, and the resulting shaming and blaming. That keeps you in a vicious cycle and takes extra effort to pull yourself back up from falling into a negative mindset yet once again. Then you have to muster up energy to cheerlead yourself back to being positive once more, believing you're worth it.

If you haven't rid your environment of junk food at home, now is the time to do it. If it's not there, you can't eat it. You have enough triggers in life without creating more. Because triggers are everywhere, you need to find a strategy to deal with them.

It's important to recognize your triggers. Are you tired due to lack of sleep? Are you feeling sad or rejected? What about being misunderstood? Make your list on page 31 in your journal under Triggers. What seems to trip you up? Be as honest as you can. This can be a working list where you can add more as you encounter them.

Now that you have made your list, think of other things you can do to either handle your emotions to not give in to self-soothing with food or to manage the food temptation. Make your list of better ways to cope with the temptation list under Actions Instead.

Now that you have both lists, you can correlate them to be a useful reference in overcoming the temptation to give in to short-term gratification. Many of the "Actions Instead" can be used for a variety of the "Triggers." You can mix and match with what is appropriate at the time. Refer to your lists often, especially "Actions Instead."

In the process of changing your mind to change your body, we have looked at recognizing your strengths with opportunities to improve your weaknesses, believing you deserve to have the body image that matches your self-image. When you fall, you will pick yourself up and reframe your negative thoughts that come with your momentary failures (they don't define you unless you let them). You'll let go of them and repeat this process until you catch yourself at the beginning of the cycle, and your first thoughts go to managing the triggers at the outset instead of giving in.

We must raise our level of awareness because our eating can be mindless, and we become aware AFTER the fact.

When you have food cravings and you overeat, take time to figure out why. *Pay close attention to how you were feeling at the time of mindlessly comforting yourself with food. What caused the pattern to start? Conflict with a friend or loved one? Feeling disrespected? Feeling disappointed? Feeling rejected? Lonely? Frustrated? Sad? Disgusted? Fearful? Hopeless? Embarrassed? Guilty? Nervous? Bored? Insecure? Exhausted? Resentful? Add these to your list of Triggers and use some of the Actions Instead or come up with ways to manage each one of these emotions. Add these to your list of Triggers and Actions Instead on page 31 in your journal.*

> We must raise our level of awareness ... and we become aware AFTER the fact.

How can we manage our emotions? Journaling helps. Choosing to pursue what makes us happy helps. We improve our emotions by how we choose to think about the situation. We see the positives and let the negatives go. If we can't change our circumstances, then we have to change our attitudes about the circumstances. As an example, you have to scrub the kitchen floor, but you don't want to. You grumble, "I don't want to clean this floor; I'm tired. Why do I have to do it? Can't someone else do it?" Or you look at it differently with, "I may not like cleaning the kitchen floor, but I'll get some good exercise; I'll feel better when it's clean, and I'll have a sense of accomplishment." You can change the

"I have to" to "I have the opportunity to." If you change your mindset to be more positive more of the time, you lessen your emotional responses to being triggered by food. This awareness has to become automatic. We are so used to reacting that we never stop to be aware of our surroundings, our emotions, and our triggers. We react and then we become aware. By then it's too late.

We react and then we become aware. By then it's too late.

You have identified how the pattern started. How will you rewrite the story so it plays out differently next time? How will you be more aware to make better choices with a previously thought-through plan?

Think about the following scenario. You go to a party and eat more than you should of all the wrong foods. Later that night, you indulge in a serving of self-hatred, shame, guilt, anger, and end up feeling depressed. You know the drill: "I'm a fat pig." "I have no discipline." "I fail at everything I do." Instead, you change the monologue to: "I messed up. It doesn't define me." "I can do better next time." "This is a marathon, and there will be bumps along the way, but I can get back up and run to the finish line." Which feels better? Which describes you? Which one would you rather have describe you?

The process doesn't end there. You need to visualize how you want to rewrite the story for next time. Will you choose happiness in being successful in your goals instead of feeling deprived over what you're giving up? Will you empower yourself with having an enjoyable time at a party which doesn't have to depend on what goes into your mouth? What about all the wonderful conversations you can have with others when you aren't hovering over the food tables? At the end of the evening, you go home without guilt or self-deprecation and are happy that you had a great time socializing. Part of the rewriting of the story is to visualize the plan you have worked out ahead of time to give you a better outcome. You have a plan, and you use it! This new approach doesn't happen by accident. You're being intentional, and it works.

What if you didn't follow your plan as you had hoped, being propelled into the same old patterns? Instead of continuing with negative self-talk, try something else. They say the definition of insanity is doing the same thing over and over, expecting different results. Instead of continuing in this negative demeaning pattern of self-betrayal, why not forgive yourself and let it go? Forgiveness is not saying what you did was okay; it's taking your power back to become the person you want to be. If you don't forgive yourself, those thoughts and actions continue to have power over you, maybe not consciously, but subconsciously. Say, "I refuse to be locked in a bond with my poor decisions regarding food and the resulting emotional devastation and dwelling on my failures. I let them go, I withdraw my emotion, and I refuse to invest in it anymore. I am free to become the person I want to be."

Forgiveness is a gift you give to yourself. You can make new choices and live in the present, starting afresh. The past is over, and you can create your future, one step at a time. The present is your gift to yourself to begin again to carve out a new way of being.

You must forgive yourself; you are more than the mistakes you have made. Part of your remorse comes from not living up to your own expectations of who you want to be. You have a choice to either wallow in self-pity or choose to become who you want to be, starting from this time forward.

Will you make mistakes and fall into old patterns? Probably. The sooner you can break the pattern and get back on track, the better. You will see more and more success and less of these patterns of defeating behaviors.

Not forgiving yourself keeps you locked up in your own emotional "prison" where you give up your dreams and hopes of being free and happy, of becoming who you want to be. The only one keeping you in prison is you. You are the one who has to open the prison door. The key is on the inside, and you're the only one who has it. No one else can unlock it for you. You have to do it; there's no other way.

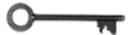

You've made the decision to take the key to unlock your prison door. You swing it open and you walk out into your new life! How will you feel? Will there be a smile on your face? Will you have a sense of relief? You can have a newfound peace and contentment. It's yours for the taking!

When you forgive yourself, you get right back into your plan of healthy living with getting enough sleep, exercising, and eating with a positive outlook of taking your power back. You choose healthier food and exercise and align your current identity with a new and improved body, which will yield positive results of more energy, feeling confident, and being happier.

This will be the process you will use over and over again. Before long you will have longer times in between failures and the need to *reframe, rewrite,* and *reconcile* by forgiving yourself. You will recognize the pattern sooner to get back on track.

Imagine doing this or some version of this to rewrite your story. We need to retrain our minds, so we automatically believe that we're worth it and we deserve better; we don't tear ourselves down when we fail, but we reframe the positives about who we are and visualize new ways of behaving around food.

When you are compassionate toward yourself, you will begin to heal. If you had a best friend who just blew it, what would you say to him or her? I'm guessing you would tell your best friend that everyone makes mistakes, that you believe in them, and they can do better next time. You need to be your own best friend and do the same for yourself!

Forgiveness empowers you to move forward with your life.

After you've forgiven yourself, you realize that we're all fallible and make wrong choices at times; it doesn't have to define you. It's okay not to be perfect. It makes us more vulnerable and more "human" to others who don't want to compare themselves to our "perfection," which is a myth.

You need to decide how you will move forward in a positive way to create the future you want to have instead of trying to fix the past, which cannot be fixed. You can put your efforts into making your life what you want it to be. Forgiveness empowers you to move forward with your life.

In the next chapter, we will discuss how we get in our own way and how we let others sabotage our goals. It's an easy trap to fall into unless we are aware of it and take steps against it. Let's continue the journey...

Chapter 10:
Danger Ahead: Watch Out for Sabotage!

"Why did I place my appetite for food before my appetite for life?"—Davina Chessid, *Food Crazy Mind*

Have you ever done something and later asked yourself, "What was I thinking?" Cindy can relate. She was invited to a birthday party, but she was reluctant to go because she knew she would be tempted with all the yummy foods. She promised herself she would be good, that she would eat healthy foods to stay on her eating plan to lose weight. Before she knew it, she had some birthday cake with ice cream on the side. Not just a small piece, but a big piece with *a lot* of ice cream. "How did that happen?" she wondered later and began her pattern of self-loathing and disgust.

We have fallen into these traps at one time or another. She didn't want to hurt the host's feelings, and she wanted to fit in socially. Cindy rationalized, saying she could start tomorrow because, after all, it's her birthday. Maybe she wanted the short-term gratification and didn't think about her long-term goals.

Do you see yourself losing weight, or is it just a dream you wish for? If everyone else (or a lot of your friends or colleagues) is overweight, you may feel there's not a strong reason to lose the weight and get healthy. You've lived with this weight for years, maybe even decades. Why change? You fit right in, your friends accept you as you are, you love food, and you're used to celebrating and comforting yourself with food. This is what you know, and you're comfortable with it.

If you're truly serious about losing weight, you must know there's no good time to start. There will always be a reason to make food a central part of the activities you attend— birthday parties, get-togethers, eating out, tailgate parties, you name it, food will be there, and we're not talking about raw vegetables and fruit. The food we celebrate with is laden with sugar and fat, which is not going to be kind to our waistlines.

On the other hand, any time is a good time to start. Once you have a plan in place and have determined you will be successful because you desire and deserve to be healthy, you can start any time, even Thanksgiving or Christmas. You don't need to wait until after the holidays or other celebrations when you may have gained more weight. You can start now!

Let's look at what might trip you up, so you can be aware of these traps and be more successful in this journey.

Sabotaging Behaviors

Sabotaging behaviors can be defined as anything we do or don't do that prevents us from reaching our goals and what we desire in life. It's the little voice in our heads that cries out to undermine our attempts to create what we desire. It cries out that "I'm not good enough," or "I don't deserve my dreams," and we rationalize to make it so. Perhaps you can relate to some of the following behaviors:

- avoidance
- not applying for a job you want
- not opting for something because you believe you don't deserve it
- procrastination on what is important to you
- not facing your fears for something better
- not making your wants and needs known
- not reaching out for what you want, whether it's a new relationship or a promotion at work
- not putting in the time and effort to learn what you need to know
- putting yourself in front of temptation when it's not in your best interest
- giving in to social pressure

How Does Sabotage Play Itself Out?

We often use rigidity as a form of self-sabotage. Refer to Chapter 7 to review all-or-nothing thinking. A person who's rigid remains set in his way without being able to see a situation from another perspective. He can't imagine saying "no" and taking a different course of action.

We self-sabotage when we have to get our needs met through others or other external means, such as food. This happens because we have not developed our own inner resources to take care of ourselves, according to Marilyn J. Sorensen, Ph.D., author of *Breaking the Chain of Low Self-Esteem*.[1]

In this process, we're not being true to ourselves. We're not standing up for ourselves or communicating our desires. We meet others' wants and needs, or what we think their expectations of us are, at our own expense.

Have you been out with friends socially when you really want to stay on your eating plan? Then come the snide comments and remarks and prodding for you to join them in what they're having. Do you give in to be socially accepted by your friends, or do you stand your ground, being true to yourself?

What has just happened in this scenario is what we call "leveling." If a person doesn't feel good about who they are or what they're doing, they try to bring you to their level. Could they have felt bad about their own struggles with food, and by getting you to join them, they have temporary relief from their own conflicts? If we give in, then we're accepted and don't have to fear making a mistake or fear rejection. This placates our anxiety for the time being at the expense of having a lot of frustration and disappointment for not taking care of our own needs.

What if you stood your ground? You don't really know what their reaction would be. Maybe they want you to "enjoy" the good-tasting food with them, but when they see your resolve, the socializing continues without a hitch. It really isn't as big of a deal as you might think it is. At the end of the evening, you will go home feeling good about following through on your decision. You're nurturing your inner resources, being your own best friend!

Why Do I Allow Sabotaging Behaviors?

What are some of the reasons we sabotage ourselves? We may be used to failure, and that's our comfort zone. If we don't perform well, we don't have to live up to higher expectations. It may be more comfortable living with the status quo than making changes, even if it's not in our best interest. Bad habits of overeating (and other vices) keep us locked into these patterns of self-sabotage. We will address habits later in Chapter 11.

We want short-term gratification and go on a binge at the expense of long-term goals. "I want what I want when I want it" is your go-to behavior. Have you considered what delaying gratification of a small reward for long-term benefit of a larger reward could do for you? Let's look at the Stanford Marshmallow Experiment.

The Stanford Marshmallow Experiment

This experiment was conducted in the 1960s and 1970s at Stanford University to explore the impact of delayed gratification vs. short-term gratification. The study looked at the strategies four-year olds used to resist temptation. They were each given one marshmallow or other such treat with two options: 1) they could have the one marshmallow at any time they wanted or 2) they could wait for the experimenter to return (in about 15 minutes—a long time for a four-year old) and then have two marshmallows for their patience. The four-year olds were faced with a *small reward now* or a *bigger reward later*. Some gave in to eat the one marshmallow whereas others were able to wait for their two marshmallows.[2]

What the researchers discovered was that the children who were able to postpone getting their two marshmallows used "cool" distraction techniques. They found ways to distract themselves by covering their eyes from looking at the marshmallow, by hiding under the table, by singing songs, or by thinking of the marshmallow as something with no taste, such as a cotton ball.

The children who used distraction methods were reevaluated as teenagers and adults. They had higher SAT scores, better social skills, self-esteem, and self-worth. They were more mature, could handle stress better, and could plan ahead and reason better. As adults, they were less likely to have drug problems or other addictions, be divorced, or be overweight, according to the study.

What was necessary for these positive outcomes to happen? There had to be the ability to bypass short-term reward for a higher payoff in the future. Being able to delay gratification also helped them with being sensitive to rejection. This increased their resolve against sabotage from others. If the four-year olds were sensitive to rejection, but were able to delay gratification, as teens and adults, they had higher self-esteem and better coping skills than those who were sensitive to rejection and who did not delay gratification. The ability to delay gratification resulted in improved functioning across time into adulthood.

There had to be the ability to bypass short-term reward for a higher payoff in the future.

What can we learn from this that will help us with our weight loss goals? First and foremost, there must be a goal you want to reach. There must be a "why." When you know your "why," that is the greater reward you're looking for. You have to desire your future and goal of health, fitness, and happiness MORE than you want that momentary pleasure.

When you do, you will find ways to not cave in to temptation. That will be your motivating force in your efforts.

Take some time now to list the "whys" for your weight loss. Go to page 33 in your journal to revisit your reasons to lose weight and keep it off. You can use your list from page 10. At this point, you may have thought of more whys, which you can add. While you are on this page, think of some "cooling" strategies you can use to avoid sabotaging the "whys" of your long-term goals.

What can you learn from these children regarding temptation? They were able to find a way within themselves to deal with the temptation. They *desired* the greater reward *more* than the immediate satisfaction of the one marshmallow. There is an expression, "You gotta have the 'want-to.'" This means your motivation is so great that it propels your desire into action. Is your desire greater than the temptation in front of you? If so, what will you do to ensure you reap your ultimate reward? What "cooling" strategies can you use? At a party, will you get your healthy food choices and leave the food table to mingle with others? Will you visualize the forbidden foods as a war zone with the resulting devastation? Could you substitute something else for it in your mind that is unappealing and could easily be resisted?

Have you thought about what you will say to well-meaning friends who tell you, "A little bit won't hurt"? What they may not realize is that it may start you down a path of unhealthy eating, just as the alcoholic cannot have one drink without eventually getting wasted.

What about a spouse or a good friend who sabotages your efforts to keep the status quo? When one person begins to change, it changes the dynamics of the relationship. It's like a tug of war. When one side pulls the rope, the other side has no choice but to move or to let go. A husband might be afraid of losing his wife if she becomes more attractive and other men become interested in her. He might need to lose a few pounds himself to keep up with her. With friends, they might not like what they see in themselves compared to the "new you" and may sabotage your efforts to keep the relationship intact.

How Do I Stop Self-Sabotaging Behavior?

Oftentimes, we aren't aware sabotaging behavior is happening. The first step you must take is to recognize when it does happen. It's easy to be aware of it after the fact, but then it's too late. You must develop a conscious awareness of what you're thinking and feeling and what your response will be to your thoughts and feelings.

At times there's a little voice in our head that tries to undermine the positive goals we seek to achieve by telling us we aren't good enough or worthy. It becomes a rationalization (rational lie) to thwart our best intentions.

It's helpful to personify the saboteur in you. When you can externalize it, you can talk back to Mr. or Mrs. Saboteur, and your self-sabotage has less power over you. Try it! It really helped me to externalize my anxiety when I was taking licensing exams.

Meditation can help you become attuned to your inner thoughts and feelings. Journaling can help untangle your thoughts about your fears, things you're uncertain about, uncomfortable feelings, and anything that could be holding you back. As you write about your thoughts and feelings, you may be surprised by the answers that are deep down inside you.

It's important to find clarity and insight about the outcomes you want to create and the potential triggers that could set you back.

Tips to Avoid Sabotaging Behaviors

- Know your "why," both as your payoff and, better yet, your motivation to gain control of your weight struggles.

- Have a go-to plan when faced with emotional struggles instead of resorting to food.

- Let go of your past to claim your future.

- Claim your right to get back in control of your life. It's time to end your struggles with weight.

- Instead of being the victim, become the victor!

- Go from being your own saboteur to becoming your own best friend and cheerleader!

In Summary

Be aware that sabotage of your weight-loss efforts will come from many places. You must be on guard as a warrior prepared for battle. Do you have a plan in place (offense) and strategies to deal with being derailed (defense) and a plan to get back on track (offense)?

In the next chapter, we will look at how creating new habits will keep us on track and change our patterns of behavior.

We will look at the anatomy of habits, our belief in them, finding a support system, and how this will be key in changing how we manage our weight-loss efforts.

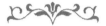

Chapter 11:
Habits Will Make You or Break You!

"Sow a thought, reap an action; sow an action, reap a habit;
sow a habit, reap a character; sow a character,
reap a destiny."
—Stephen R. Covey, *The 7 Habits of Highly Effective People*

Habits! We all have them. Some are good, and others are just bad. We can rattle off a myriad of bad habits, and we stretch to find the good ones. We fall into bad habits because we succumb to the easiest course of action. We give in to our feelings and to what feels good in the moment, but at a later cost. This can be anything from procrastinating and not getting that report done to watching TV and not getting the dishes done or laundry piling up to, "Oops, I had that piece of cake" and derailing our weight-loss efforts. It's *so* easy to give in to what we want, to what feels good in the moment; it takes work to align ourselves with what's in our best interests and the ultimate rewards we're looking for.

We have habits we're not even aware of, routines of behaviors on a regular basis that become automatic. We get up in the morning to go to work, brush our teeth, make coffee, get dressed, and get ready for the day. When we get to work, we greet the boss, do our work, and, at the end of the day, prepare to go home. When we arrive home, we greet our family; if you're single, you may turn on music or the TV or call a friend. These are habits that happen without thought; they've become automatic routines and stand us in good stead.

Bad habits are hard to break, and good habits take time to become part of our daily experience. Our bad habits have been imprinted in our neural pathways, but we can form new good habits through repetition.[1] When we repeatedly continue a behavior, we increase the link between the context and the action.[2] This improves the automatic nature of behavior for that context. We will know when a behavior is automatic when we're not aware of it and we're no longer being intentional to make it happen.[3]

In Charles Duhigg's *The Power of Habit*, he describes the formation of habits. Automatic habits have a cue, a routine, and a reward. Take, for instance, brushing your teeth. You have just eaten and know there's food residue left in your mouth. That's the cue. Then you brush (and floss)—the routine. The reward is having fresh breath and clean teeth and gums. In going to work, the cue is the Monday, Tuesday, Wednesday, Thursday, or Friday when you're scheduled for work. Unless you have a reason to get up on Saturday or Sunday, you may or may not set your alarm. The routine is setting your alarm (Monday through Friday) and getting up when it goes off to get ready for work. The reward is your paycheck to pay your bills, and if you love your job, fulfillment and social interaction.[4]

We also have bad habits that don't serve us well. You may have a habit when you come home (cue), you grab a bite to eat when you're not hungry (routine), which relieves some stress from the day (reward). The cues and the rewards remain the same. What if you changed the routine? Instead of grabbing a bite to eat when you're *not* hungry, what if you played with your dog or got some ice water with lemon and sat down, either with your spouse or alone, and de-stressed.

On page 35 in your journal, think about new habits to put in place that will make you successful. Keep the cue and reward the same, but change the routine.

A Powerful Illustration of Habit

Creating good habits can be very powerful. Would you believe changing the routine while keeping the cue and reward intact, could lead to a Super Bowl victory? That's how powerful it is!

The following is a summary of Tony Dungy's journey as described in Charles Duhigg's *The Power of Habit*.4 His coaching philosophy was to train his team by making their plays to be automatic habits, over and over; there was no last minute reactive decision that could cost them the play. It would become so habitual that the other team would have no time to react.

Instead of changing the whole habit, he changed the routine with the cue and reward remaining intact, remaining familiar. If you keep the cue and reward the same, changing the routine will change the habit.

Dungy took a job in 1996 with the Tampa Bay Buccaneers using his coaching philosophy. Over the next few years, the Bucs' record continued to improve and before long, they were a viable contending team, but something was happening when the pressure was on. They were falling apart; they were resorting to their old comfort zone, to what they had always done, and it wasn't working. After blowing critical games in the playoffs three years in a row, players said they were "going back to what we knew." Although they said they trusted the system of relying on their well-practiced habits, they resorted to what was comfortable when under pressure. They didn't really believe all the way to the end. Result: Dungy was fired, but the Buccaneers went on to win the Super Bowl the following year using his methods.

The Need for Belief in Sustaining Habits

Belief is the necessary ingredient that makes a new habit into a permanent behavior.

Habit replacement works until a stressful event enters the picture. The difference with those who make it and those who don't is belief. Belief is the necessary ingredient that makes a new habit into a permanent behavior. There has to be the belief that change is possible.

Coach Dungy was offered a position with the Indianapolis Colts. Although the Colts qualified for the playoffs, the same problems were emerging as they had in Tampa Bay. Under the stress of the playoffs, the Colts went back to their comfort zones and their old habits rather than believing in the new habits that gave them a winning record to get to the playoffs.

Tony Dungy faced tragedy with his son's suicide. The Colts lost their first playoff game that season. Over the course of time, the team watched Dungy's reactions in handling tragedy. The Colts rallied and something changed. The team bonded with their coach and began to catch his vision for playing the game. They began to believe; they became a team, not just 11 players on the field playing football, but a team that was committed to the vision of their coach. As a team, they inspired each other into believing their new vision.

In 2006, the Indianapolis Colts, with their newfound belief in their coach's vision, made it to the playoffs. They won their first playoff game and then took the divisional title. The next hurdle was the conference championship, which Dungy had lost *eight* times before. The Colts had to *believe* to overcome the Patriots, and they did, *finally*. They went on to win the Super Bowl. Everything they had learned carried through in the most stressful times because they *finally believed* and implemented their well-practiced habits.

Alcoholics Anonymous

An organization that has made good use of changing routines in forming new habits and providing supportive belief is Alcoholics Anonymous (AA). What has made AA so successful? Instead of attacking the biochemical issues of alcoholism, AA looks at the *habits* around the alcohol use. Even the most difficult habits can be changed. (This includes habits of the food addict, which we will get to later.) Although AA is not based on academics, its success and solid foundation is based on how habits are created and maintained: the cue, routine, and reward. If a member of AA looks at the cues and rewards that encourage his drinking, he can find new routines, keeping the cues and rewards, to change his behavior. You may have heard of the expression for alcoholics and drug addicts that they need to change "people, places, and things." The cues and rewards remain the same, but by changing the routine of "people, places, and things," new behaviors are created that work for the addict. It's a matter of changing the routine from the trigger, keeping the reward intact.

Just as AA has had success with helping alcoholics conquer their addictions, we, too, can look at changing the routine of the habit cycle. Overeaters Anonymous (OA) is based on AA's principles and can be very helpful in making necessary changes. What if we adopt the same routine changes that AA and OA do with changing people, places, and things? What would this look like for you? Would you change where you go to eat and find friends with healthier eating lifestyles? What about having a hobby or something you're passionate about to replace your desire to mindlessly eat? How will you implement belief in your new habits?

On page 36 in your journal, think about what you can change as your routine to give yourself more success.

Another Illustration of Habit Change and Belief

When I was in high school, the student who sat behind me in math class said he always wanted to write a book when he grew up. I had no interest.

As I grew up and had many life experiences, i.e., living in Jordan and war-torn Beirut, I wrote about them in newsletters home to family and friends. People commented on my writing and encouraged me to continue. After getting married and having four children, I wanted to share the information in written form, but there was one problem. I could say what I wanted to say in two to three pages. How could I write a book?

That was my dilemma. How could I write enough material to create a whole book? Yet, deep down inside I wanted to.

How did this dream become a reality? Not long ago, I listened to some presentations on self-publishing. I asked myself, "If I don't try to do this now with help being offered in the process, when would I?" I didn't want to have any regrets; I took the plunge!

The plan was laid out ahead of us. We were to write, write, write, until our rough draft was completed. This took setting up the habit of writing every day—30 to 60 minutes—before work. What I soon discovered was the Self-Publishing School community was supportive and helpful. They helped me believe I could do this, and I supported them in their efforts. Together as a group, we are believing, supporting each other, and making it happen!

In Summary

You can dissect your habits to see why you respond to your cues with the resulting rewards. Replacing the existing routine with a new one will result in getting the reward in a more productive way. Along with changing the routine, it's important to find a group with the same goals and beliefs for accountability and support. Now would be a good time to find some friends who struggle with their weight, download the free journal, and get together for support. When you commit your goals to a group, you improve your odds for success dramatically. Being part of a group inspires belief and change, even if it's only one other person. Go for it!

The same can be true for you in your weight-loss efforts. Maybe you've tried before but haven't been successful, or you lost the weight but went back to sloppy eating habits. If you will follow the principles in this book and find a support group or create one of your own, I promise you that you will make this happen!

If I could show a logical progression, it would look something like this:

Information → Application (Cue, Routine, Reward) → Support and Accountability → Belief → Continued Application = Weight-Loss Success!

There has to be the belief that change is possible. This change and belief is facilitated in the context of a group with the same values and vision. Please stay tuned for Chapter 12 on accountability, both personal and in a group, to solidify making belief and change possible!

Here's an example of habit change that I think you will enjoy:

PORTRAIT OF PROGRESS

By Portia Nelson

Chapter 1: "I walk down the street. There is a deep hole in the sidewalk. I fall in. I am lost ... I am helpless. It isn't my fault. It takes forever to find a way out."

Chapter 2: "I walk down the same street. There is a deep hole in the sidewalk. I pretend I don't see it. I fall in again. I can't believe I am in the same place, but it isn't my fault. It still takes a long time to get out."

Chapter 3: "I walk down the same street. There is a deep hole in the sidewalk. I see it is there. I still fall in ... it's habit. My eyes are open. I know where I am. It is my fault. I get out immediately."

Chapter 4: "I walk down the same street. There is a deep hole in the sidewalk. I walk around it."

Chapter 5: "I walk down another street."

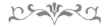

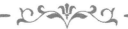

Chapter 12:
Accountability: It's Up to Me!

"If it is to be, it's up to me."—Lolly Daskal

You may say, "If it's up to me, why do I need accountability?" Let's consider what the term *accountability* means and what it entails.

Accountability can be defined as being liable, answerable, or responsible for. It means we have an obligation to report, explain, or justify our actions. We are responsible and have to answer to the results we get or don't get. This can include accountability to ourselves, to another person, or to a group of people with the same purpose.

As mentioned above, two kinds of accountability are important—group and personal accountability. Let's look at personal accountability first.

Personal Accountability

Accountability starts with you! It's being responsible from within, holding yourself accountable.

Another way of looking at accountability is to think of it as delivering on a commitment. We're responsible for an outcome—our weight loss—with that as the goal in mind. This requires daily follow-through to get the results we desire in the end.

With accountability, we make and keep our promise, or we must give an account as to why it didn't happen. We must then problem-solve and implement a plan, so it doesn't happen again in the future.

When we make right choices, we grow and feel good about ourselves. It improves our self-esteem because we are proud of being true to our integrity. We live up to who we want to become. If we don't follow through with making good choices, it wears away at the very fiber of our being.

Making right choices comes from the very core of who we are. It takes courage and believing in ourselves. We must make our decisions in the

We live up to who we want to become.

here-and-now to avoid our own sabotaging behaviors and those from others, to be true to our values and what we desire.[1]

Our accountability stems from the daily choices we make, whether we give in to short-term gratification or have the courage to say no, keeping our greater goals in mind.

Components of Personal Responsibility

Here are some factors to consider, helping you be accountable with your weight-loss goals:

Clear Expectations

It's important to have clear (and realistic) expectations. It's easier to measure, and you know your target. Summarize your action steps by saying them out loud (this helps with commitment) and by writing them down.

Have an Accountability Contract that you will sign and date. Keep it posted where you will see it and be reminded of your commitment to lose weight in order to gain better health, energy, and happiness. *See page 41 in your journal.*

Clear Capability/Preparation

Ask yourself if you have what's necessary to be successful in your weight-loss journey.

- Do you have a food scale (if you need one)?
- What about scales to weigh yourself or a tape measure?
- Do you have an eating lifestyle plan picked out? (See Chapter 13)
- Does your plan fit with your personality style? (See Chapter 13)

Clear Way to Measure

Do you have weekly milestones with measurable results?

- How many pounds do you want to lose?
- Do you see an increase in energy?
- Are you getting more sleep?
- Are you lowering your stress levels?

If you're not meeting your goals, look at what's getting in your way. Do you get enough sleep? Are you comfort eating? Is tempting food lying out, and you can't resist? Now is your time to troubleshoot and think of some solutions to put in place. If your goal is unreasonable, you need to redefine it to be more achievable to get back on track.

Here are some questions to ask yourself to problem-solve any slip-ups you may have had:

- *How can I get my eating, exercise, sleep, and stress management back on track?*
- *What was my contribution to the problem, instead of blaming others?*
- *What can I do to keep this from happening again?*

Think of ways you have let yourself down with the above questions and record your answers on page 38 in your journal.

Clear Feedback

It's important to frequently evaluate your progress. You can do this by weighing once a week, using your tape measure, or both. Ask yourself if you're on track. If you are, great! If there's a problem, can you explain why? For instance, if you have had a stressful week, that could account for not losing, or even gaining a little, even if you have been true to your diet plan and exercising. Recognize normal plateaus, and don't lose heart. If you were at fault for not meeting your goal, figure out what went wrong, so you can make some course corrections.

Accountability with a Friend or a Group

According to Peter Bregman, when you share your dreams and goals with a friend or in a group, you're partnering together for the success of each other. You provide support and belief that together you can do this, that you desire to do this, and that you need each other's support and encouragement. There is mutual accountability; everyone gives an account of their week's success or difficulties. You can also find accountability with a friend who may not need to lose weight, but who will keep you accountable, and you can return the favor for something they're struggling with.

There is power collectively as a group. When you see others being successful, you know it's possible to lose weight, and you will be able to do it, too. When you see someone struggling, you know you're not alone. At this point, a group can be very supportive and understanding while holding you accountable to your intentions and goals. If others are firm to help you to not rationalize your mistakes, this is the time to be thankful, not hurt by their firmness.[2]

Components of Having a Group that Works

When you set up your group, have some ground rules for everyone. Here are a few from Bregman that are standard to get you started. Feel free to add more that are important to you.

- Confidentiality is the foundation for your group. What is shared in the group stays in the group.

- Be honest. You can't make progress if you're not forthcoming with the truth.

- Do not give advice unless it's asked for.

- Accept each other's journey.

- Listen, and give everyone a chance to share.

- Avoid having side conversations; it's disrespectful to the one sharing.
- No cell phones or other electronic devices.
- Be supportive and encouraging to others.
- Be on time; be respectful of each other.

One of the reasons AA has been successful is because those who attend meetings feel understood and can get help to get back on the wagon. They know they're not alone and help is only a meeting away. (If you find you're struggling with food addiction, you can check out Overeaters' Anonymous. They use the 12-step principles that AA uses.)

That's what meeting with a friend or a group can do for you. You're in it together, you understand where each one is coming from, and there's acceptance. In the group, you can share your success or failure, find support, find encouragement, help someone else figure out how to get back on track, and together believe you can do this! It will fuel the fire!

... will you create a happy, victorious life with celebration? The choice is yours!

Accountability, whether as an individual, with a group or with a friend, helps. Ultimately, you're the only one who can rewrite the story of your life. Will it be a sad ending that results in failure to lose weight, or will you create a happy, victorious life with celebration? The choice is yours!

With your own expectations and commitments in place, along with having support from a friend or a group, you're ready to move forward. In the next section, you'll get started with an eating plan that's right for you (you decide, so you'll have ownership) and the trifecta of proper sleep, stress management, and exercise. They all go hand-in-hand and affect each other, as you will see when you read the following chapters. Let's get to the heart of what you'll be doing.

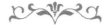

THE PLAN

Chapter 13:
Where Do I Start?

"Do or do not. There is no TRY."—Yoda, *Star Wars*

Isn't it a good feeling to be at this point in your journey to lose weight and keep it off? No more yo-yo dieting! You've done a lot of hard work! You've looked at your self-worth, patterns you've fallen into that sabotage you over and over again; you're reclaiming your right to take control of negative thoughts and longstanding patterns that hold you hostage. It's time to begin a lifestyle that will create the life of happiness and contentment you desire and deserve to have to live your best life. It's time to break free!

Food Preferences and Lifestyle Choices

First of all, you need to assess your food preferences and lifestyle choices to pick a program that will work for you. Would counting points as with Weight Watchers be too cumbersome, or would it be "just the thing," giving you a structure to follow and flexibility in eating out? Would you prefer to count calories? What about no carbs? Or no fat? Or portion control? I have listed some popular diets to get you started in your research. This will help you take ownership of whatever plan you decide to follow.

Personality Preferences
What is My Myers-Briggs Type Indicator?

This section is optional. It gives you insight in how you react around food. It's really fun to get to know yourself better with this tool. I highly recommend that you go to *humanmetrics.com* and/or *16personalities.com* and go through the process to find out your type. If you're interested in gaining a better understanding of your type and what makes you "tick," you can read, *Type Talk: The 16 Personality Types That Determine How We Live, Love, and Work,* by Otto Kroeger and Janet M. Thuesen.

Otto Kroeger specializes in the Myers-Briggs Type Indicator (MBTI) and has made some observations regarding type and dieting. This is not research-based yet, just observations he has made. See if it makes sense for your personality style.

Extraversion (E) and Introversion (I)

Extraverts may have a harder time losing weight because they naturally respond to their environment and love to be with people. This sets them up for more socializing around food. Because of their outward focus, they're less aware of their eating habits. Taking a picture of his/her plate of food helps an extravert keep up with how much is being consumed.

Introverts, on the other hand, are more aware of what they're eating due to their "inner attentiveness." Journaling may work better for introverts because they process internally.

Either way, keeping track of what you're eating is a valuable tool to help in holding yourself accountable.

Sensing (S) and iNtuitive (N)

If you're a Sensing (S) type, you may experience weight-loss success a little more easily than your iNtuitive (N) friends do. Sensors are more attuned to their senses and can enjoy food without overeating. The N's finish their plate of food and go back for more because they didn't take the time to enjoy it while they were eating it.

Another difference between S's and N's is their concept of "here-and-now" for the S and "tomorrow" for the N. If an N fails on a diet today, there will always be tomorrow, since they're future thinkers. Conceptually, an iNtuitive may think, "That was good; imagine what more would be like."

Could an iNtuitive benefit from Sensing habits? Probably. It may be difficult to sustain. An iNtuitive's best bet would be to try one of the other approaches, watching out for iNtuition getting in the way.

Thinking (T) and Feeling (F)

Feelers (F) have a harder time with losing weight than do Thinkers (T) for a number of reasons. Since F's are relational, food presents the opportunity for having intimacy and harmony with others. Food is often used by Feelers for comfort and as a reward. A Thinker would not necessarily use food as a reward, since the Thinker is logical and "I expected myself to be good," as Otto Kroeger puts it.

Relationships are important to an F, and they want to please others. This makes it even more difficult beyond giving in to the temptation presented to the F. They find it difficult to say "No" to family, friends, and a party host. If a friend comes into town, it is difficult to turn down having a meal together.

Because of their tendency to please people, they find it difficult to ask for what they want in a restaurant (potential to cause disharmony) and to disappoint a date by not having dessert.

Feelers can benefit by having a good support system in their efforts to lose weight, and they need to make others aware of their weight-loss goals. Thinkers are logical about their goals of weight loss. If they slip up, they can more easily get back on track to accomplish their goals. They don't lose a lot of emotional energy over slip-ups, whereas F's can benefit from having extra support to get back on track.

Judgers (J) and Perceivers (P)

Judgers (J) go to closure on making a decision as a judge decides a case. Perceivers (P) like to "go with the flow" and are spontaneous. J's have an easier time with weight loss because they set goals and find motivation in achieving those goals. They also like structure and are good at planning.

Judgers have a built-in sense of being in control and know when they're out of control. A Perceiver, on the other hand, is more spontaneous and has a lower sense of control. A P can impulsively wake up one morning and decide to go on a diet whereas a J will plan which day to start and will prepare to have all necessary foods and items ready and available to begin.

If P's try to force themselves into a J diet, they will fail repeatedly. They need to take it one day at a time. Instead of focusing on the goal, they could consider eating less. They will do well with a variety of diet menus available, such as high fiber, low fat, carbohydrates, frozen food, health food, vegan menus, gourmet, etc., and choose from them according to their desire at the time. This gives them freedom to be spontaneous and does not cramp their style.

Some Conclusions About Type

ISTJ's appear to have the easiest time in managing their weight. Kroeger states that the thousands of ISTJ's he has met over the years are in good physical shape. If an ISTJ is overweight, they're likely to be experiencing a stress-related problem. If you think about it, ISTJ's are better at managing their schedules to get proper sleep and exercise, which has a huge impact on weight-loss efforts.

ENFP's struggle more with their weight due to the aforementioned factors. If you find an ENFP without a weight problem, they're either dealing with a lot of stress and not eating as much, have learned how to conquer their struggle with weight loss and constantly monitor weight fluctuations, or they have a high metabolism that burns calories more readily.

How to Succeed According to Your Temperament

As we've seen, certain types struggle more with weight loss than other types. Let's see if we can tap into some of the different subtypes to see what might work for you.

The NF Diet

When an iNtuitive-Feeler (NF) decides to lose weight, they do it for the sake of a relationship they're in. They have to know there will be benefit to the relationship and what positive feedback they will get from others. They will not lose weight for themselves; they will lose weight in the context of a relationship.

If you're an NF and have a spouse or partner who loves you as you are, there will be little motivation to lose weight. Perhaps your goal could be to maintain your weight as opposed to setting goals you're unlikely to meet. If your weight is a health issue, you could rally support from your relationship for better health and longevity.

If NF's are unhappy about their weight, they may blame themselves for failure to get affirmations from others, according to Kroeger. For them, it's rarely about weight. They need to see themselves more realistically. Before even considering a weight-loss plan, it would be prudent for the NF to examine how they really look and feel.

The NF would do well by setting up a contract with someone. In the midst of shedding pounds, they can probe into their motivations and feel guilty when they fail. Unfortunately, this can lead to overeating to assuage their guilt. Their best chance of success would be tied to pleasing someone in a relationship.

The NT Diet

In this scenario, an NT (iNtuitive-Thinker) will find success in making weight loss a competition. They enjoy the challenge of self-mastery. NT's will plan their diet in their minds, but it might end there as well. For the NT, it's important to have a conceptual base, to grasp onto "the why" of needing to change.

Because NT's are involved with ideas and possibilities, they're likely to create a diet plan from two to three different diets that will meet their needs. Because they think conceptually, they take a systems approach. If they're afraid of failing, they shy away from an approach that could lead to failure.

The SJ Diet

An SJ (Sensor-Judger) finds his motivation to lose weight as being responsible. SJ's do not usually seek to please others, and their diet is not a competition; their motivation and reward is to set a goal and to accomplish it as soon as possible.

What we know about dieting relates to the SJ perspective. They value responsibility and structure and will set up a program they can successfully carry out, using lists and eating plans.

According to Kroeger, if an SJ struggles with dieting, Extraversion or Feeling attributes or both may be causing the problem.

I hope you will use this information to help you decide how you want to set up your weight-loss strategy to be successful in shedding those unwanted pounds. If you have hiccups along the way, this might help you to understand the underlying causes and give you a sense of how to make changes according to your personality style. When you understand how you function, you will be better prepared for success!

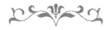

Taking Action

Making it Happen

You've done a lot of hard work! You've looked at your internal dialogues to change them to be more aligned with the "you" you desire to be. You're claiming what you deserve. You've also looked at triggers and self-sabotaging behaviors. You've made your list of triggers and "rational lies." You've also addressed fears of failure or perhaps fears of success and what could be required at a higher level of functioning.

You have a journey ahead of you. The road will have its bumps along the way, but you can do this! As Mitch Matthews, coauthor of "The Coach Mindset" program says, "Between the plan and the action...it's important to recheck the 'why.'" In your journal on page 10, review your whys to losing weight to help you stay the course.

> "Between the plan and the action...it's important to recheck the 'why.'"

Before going on any weight-loss program of diet and exercise, always consult with your doctor.

Making a Goal

You need to know what your goals are. There's a saying that if you aim at nothing, you will surely hit it. These goals should be specific to give you a clear focus for you to know when you've achieved them. Make sure you verbalize your goals with positive statements. Do you want to lose 10, 20, 50, or more pounds? Maybe you have inches to lose. Be as specific as possible. Start with weighing and measuring yourself. This is important. You will see progress if you know your starting point. Or you might have health goals—more energy, improvements in cholesterol and glucose levels, and better sleep.

With Mike Merriam's permission, think about the following as it relates to your goals:

> "What your goals ARE is less important than HOW you ENGAGE with them. It's about the LANGUAGE you use, the RESPONSES you choose, the DECISIONS you make, and the ACTIONS you take."

*On page 40 in your journal, list your goals, making sure you're moving **toward** something positive and **not away** from something negative. Write it down as your commitment to yourself; sign and date it to solidify your intent.*

Making Your Plan

Once you've decided what your goals are, you need a strategy to achieve them. You can check out various plans online. Think about what you want in a program that you believe you will have the greatest success with. You must take ownership of the plan you choose. Here's a list to get you started. There are many more out there. Find one you believe will work best for you. Make sure it will be compatible with your lifestyle and you understand the drawbacks as well.

If you go back to Chapter 2 on food addiction, look at the number you came up with when you answered the questions at the end of the chapter. The lower the number, the more flexibility you have. The higher the number, the more you will need to eliminate sugar and flour from your diet.

We can set up "bright lines" in our eating (Chapter 2). For some, it might be not having certain foods in the environment; for others, it might be the complete elimination of sugar and flour.

This list will get you started:

- The 20/20 Diet (Dr. Phil)–20 foods with thermogenic properties
- Weight Watchers (new focus on health; counting points)
- Mediterranean Diet
- Paleo Diet (good for blood pressure, weight loss, even metabolic syndrome)
- Atkins Diet (shed pounds without having to completely give up fatty foods; time sensitive)
- DASH Diet (Dietary Approaches to Stop Hypertension)–good for everyone
- TLC (Therapeutic Lifestyle Changes) Diet–also heart healthy
- Vegetarian (www.nutritionfacts.org)
- Vegan (www.nutritionfacts.org)
- South Beach Diet
- The Food Solution, by Cari Shaefer
- Bright Line Eating (Dr. Susan Peirce Thompson–no sugar or flour)

With your goals set and a plan determined, decide you're going to do this, no matter what. Don't let anything or anyone cause you to stumble. This will mean not responding to advertising, preplanning choices when eating out, and making your kitchen and office "safe" (if it's not there, you can't eat it). When you lose, and you will, get rid of your baggy clothes so you never go there again!

It takes willpower and resolve to change your habits. You change the routine of the habit (cue, routine, reward), but it takes resolve until it becomes automatic. Make sure to read the chapters on sleep, stress, and exercise which can all help you manage your willpower. Don't shortchange these areas in your life!

You need to be intentional with your new style of eating, which requires some preplanning. Part of your plan should include how much sleep and exercise you will get and how you will implement positive strategies to manage stress in your life.

Making Progress

Break your goals into small measurable steps. The task at hand won't be as overwhelming, and you can reward yourself for meeting milestones along the way. Please don't reward yourself with food!

On page 42 in your journal, make a list of rewards you can use for motivation. For women: a pedicure or manicure, some new jewelry, a new outfit or a scarf to dress up an outfit you already have (or would like to fit into), or a movie you've been wanting to see (but without the popcorn and soda). You get the idea. For men: go to a sporting event; go to a movie you've wanted to see; or buy a new shirt, sweater, or pants. Come up with things you'd like to do that don't involve food as a reward. If money is a problem, what about visiting a friend, going for a walk on the beach, going for a hike in the woods, doing a jigsaw puzzle, indulging in reading a good book you haven't had time for? Come up with some ideas that are meaningful to you.

Please don't think of losing weight as needing to take all the weight off as quickly as possible. It took a while to pack on the pounds—it will take some time to get rid of them for good. Think of your weight-loss journey as being a marathon, not a sprint. You're in it for the long haul. Once you lose your weight, you will still need to monitor triggers and instant gratification vs. long-term reward.

Making Monitoring and Accountability a Priority

You've already read the chapter on accountability. If you know you have to report to someone about how you did with your weekly goal, you will be more likely to work harder to meet it. At Weight Watchers, there is a weekly weigh-in. You don't have to go to Weight Watchers. I recommend that you set up your own group of two or more using your journal as a guide to support each other and provide accountability. If you need to, review Chapter 12.

Making a Mindset Change

You have to see yourself differently. Overweight people tend to gain more weight, not lose it, because they don't lose their plump self-image. When you lose that image and take ownership of how you want to see yourself in a new way, you will change your behaviors around food in order to maintain it.

How do you see yourself in your mind's eye?

- How do you look?

- How do you feel?

- How is your posture?

- How do you carry yourself when you walk into a room?

- Are you confident, and do you portray yourself that way?

When you can rally your emotions to get to the point that you want a better life for yourself, you will be ready! Remember our feelings drive our behaviors to lose weight. The driving force to make a decision comes from your feelings. Isn't it time for you to say, "It is my time!"

... our feelings drive our behaviors to lose weight.

Making Your Road Map for Weight-Loss Success

To summarize:

- You must have a lifestyle plan you can embrace for the long haul.

- Have mini-goals with a reward linked to their achievement. Enjoy!

- Figure out your triggers (places, times of day, people in your life, etc.) and either eliminate them or have a plan in place.

- Don't medicate your feelings with food. If you're hurting emotionally, reach out for help!

- Build your support team; build in accountability.

Remember: Losing weight and keeping it off takes effort and intention. Making a lifestyle change includes your *eating habits, exercise, sleep, stress management,* and a *mindset change* for the long haul.

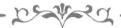

Chapter 14:
Stress—Do I Need a "Chill Pill"?

"Focus on your purpose, and your stress will melt away."
—Debasish Mridha

Stress … we all have stress! We're either working too much or making too many commitments, and we feel overwhelmed. We have families to care for, who get the leftover crumbs of our lives at times. It's as if we're on a hamster's wheel and can't get off. But we wish we could!

Stress can come from many avenues, from either external or internal sources. Let's look at them individually.

Sources of Stress

External Stressors

We're bombarded with stress in many areas. We have stress when we move, whether it's across town or across the country, with the ensuing adjustments to be made. There's work stress or school stress with their demands and impending deadlines. We take on a new job and worry about the learning curve and performance. A lot of stress can come from relationship difficulties—normal conflict or a toxic relationship. Of course, money is a big stressor in not only having enough, but also in deciding how to spend it, especially if you're in a relationship with another person (savers vs. spenders). We're doing too much with schedules that are overbooked without having any margins. There always seems to be something going on with either our spouse or children (grades, friends, overextended schedules, etc.) and our extended families.

Internal Stressors

Our internal stressors come from our own making. This is something we can control and change. Some internal stressors include worrying about everything, the "what ifs" that never happen, and those things we don't have control over. It also comes from having an all-or-nothing mindset, allowing other cognitive distortions (see Chapter 7) to rule our thinking and emotions. This causes us to be pessimistic, looking on the dark side, with negative self-chatter that's constantly trying to derail us. We're often disappointed and become angry when we have unrealistic expectations. It's imperative to become a little more flexible and understanding of the situation or the other's viewpoint.

Consider what causes stress in your life. On page 43 in your journal, list both external and internal stressors. What external stressors are causing you trouble? Can you mind-map possible solutions or directions to take? What about your internal stressors? Do you engage in too much worry or negative self-talk? If you're interested in improving in these areas, a helpful book is Dr. David Burns's The Feeling Good Handbook *(with extra chapters on communication and various common fears, even a chapter on "How to Give a Dynamic Interview When You're Scared Stiff").*[1]

Have you seen episodes of "The Biggest Loser" when, even though the contestants have done everything right with what they ate and how they exercised, they gained a couple of pounds? They attributed the weight gain to extra stress they dealt with that week.

Signs and Symptoms of Stress

Stress can manifest itself in different ways, usually either physically or psychologically. Here are some of the symptoms.

Physical Symptoms:

- Tight muscles
- Chest pressure or tightness in your chest
- Headaches
- Backaches
- Jaw tension
- Tension in your neck or shoulders
- Stomach upsets
- Insomnia
- Lack of energy
- High blood pressure
- Allergies
- Grinding your teeth at night
- Excessive perspiration
- Cold hands or feet
- Overeating

Psychological Symptoms:

- Anxiety
- Depression
- Forgetfulness
- Trouble concentrating
- Feeling overwhelmed
- Feeling hyperactive, as if you can't slow down
- Loneliness
- Relationship problems
- Unhappy with work
- Irritability
- Boredom
- Excessive worry
- Guilt from not being able to handle everything
- Sexual problems

Why Do You Need to Deal With Stress?

We need to manage stress because it affects our health, which affects everything else. It also interferes with our relationships and activities; it causes a decrease in productivity and time off work; it worsens problems we face, such as insomnia, headaches, stomach problems, anxiety, and depression. It also contributes to heart disease with increased cortisol, the stress hormone.

How Does Stress Affect Our Weight?

According to Dr. Melanie Greenberg, if we have long periods of time in which we are stressed, the following can happen— our appetites are increased, we hold onto fat more readily, our willpower to live a healthy lifestyle is diminished, and we resort to food.[2]

Let's look at the four areas where stress contributes to our weight gain:

Our Hormones

What happens to our hormones when we face threat or stress of any kind? Our brains go into action and release adrenaline, CRH (corticotrophin-releasing hormone), and cortisol, the "stress" hormone. The adrenaline helps us to feel alert and ready to handle the threat or stress, whether it's stress at work, a credit card bill, divorce papers, or the perception of physical danger. Our bodies go into action. While the adrenaline is

We have cortisol wanting us to replace energy from stress we experience, so we reach for food.

in play, we don't feel hungry because our blood is flowing away from our organs to our large muscles for "fight or flight." When the adrenaline wears off, cortisol signals our bodies to restore our food supply. This system worked well long ago for those fighting off dangers, using a lot of energy that needed to be replaced. However, the stress we face today does not use up a lot of energy. We have cortisol wanting us to replace energy from stress we experience, so we reach for food.

Belly Fat

When our ancestors had to deal with wild animals and famines, their bodies adapted by storing fat supplies to be used when needed. If we are chronically stressed, we also store body fat. What once worked for man long ago doesn't work well for us today. It would help to recognize this and make adjustments accordingly. This extra belly fat is unhealthy and hard to get rid of. It leads to inflammation, which increases our chances of having heart disease, diabetes, or other diseases. Extra cortisol slows our metabolism, which makes it harder to lose weight.

Anxiety

That restless feeling and being fidgety and agitated can lead to "stress" or "emotional" eating. Either eating too much or eating the wrong foods for comfort as a response to stress is very common. According to the American Psychological Association's (APA) "Stress in America" survey, 40% of the people who were surveyed reported emotional eating to deal with stress while 42% of the people reported watching two or more hours of television a day to manage stress. While you're being a couch potato (a sedentary lifestyle that's now called the "new smoking"), there is the temptation to couple this with eating. While you're "vegging out," you're not burning extra calories. When you're anxious, there's a tendency to eat mindlessly, eating more without enjoying what you just ate. That's no fun!

Cravings and Emotional Eating

If we're always stressed, we crave "comfort foods" (you know what your go-to-foods are—chips, sweets, ice cream, etc.). This is both a biological and psychological process. Stress interferes with our reward system in our brain, and increased cortisol can cause us to want more fat and sugar. Cortisol causes us to eat for more energy to replace what was used in our "fight" or "flight" mode with adrenaline.

According to Greenberg, when stressed, we want to calm our frazzled nerves with a drive through our favorite fast food establishment rather than going home to cook a healthy meal. Long commutes can increase our stress and decrease our willpower because we're hungrier when we get home. A simple solution is to carry a small bag of almonds or walnuts or other healthy snacks to stave off hunger, so you can make it home to cook a healthy meal.

Ways to Minimize Stress

Since we can't completely avoid stress, here are some ways to minimize it:

- Get up a few minutes earlier than your scheduled time.
- Get ready for the next day the night before.
- Don't rely on your memory; have things written down.
- Say "No" more often.
- Walk wherever you can.
- Make copies of your important papers and keep the originals in a safe place.
- Allow extra time.

How to Manage Stress

We can manage stress by changing our thinking and our actions. Our thoughts are very powerful. They affect our feelings and our actions. When we change our thoughts, our feelings improve, and we're then able to make better choices for our actions. Here are some tips:

Change my thoughts:

- View the stress as an opportunity for growth.
- Think of the positives you already have in your life.
- Adjust your expectations.
- Ask yourself, "Will this matter in a year?"
- Ask yourself, "Is this stressor really worth getting upset over?"
- Remind yourself that worrying about it won't help and will stress you more.

Change my actions:

- Slow down and do some deep breathing exercises to calm yourself to think and respond appropriately. Meditation and mindfulness can also help.
- Share your feelings with a trusted friend.
- Don't create more stress by overeating, drinking, or smoking.
- Seek advice from those who can steer you in the right direction. For example, your boss can help prioritize his expectations of your workload if you're overwhelmed with too much to do.

- Find time to de-stress by going for a walk, reading, listening to music, etc. A change of scenery can do wonders for you and can help you get a new perspective and refocus your energies.

- Create some margins in your life by setting boundaries. Don't be afraid to say "No." This can help to not overcommit yourself.

Learn Mindful Eating

Meditation can help you cope with stress and make you more aware of what you're eating. You learn to be aware of the sight, texture, and smell of the foods you're eating. You become more aware of your feeling hungry or feeling full, rather than eating just "because." This can help with binge eating and improving how you feel.

Find Activities Unrelated to Food

What are some things you enjoy doing? Do you like to hike, read a book, walk your dog, get a massage, or spend time with family and friends? Pleasurable activities, whatever they are, can reduce stress in your life. If you will make time to reduce your stress, you will be more refreshed, think more clearly, be more productive, be in a better mood, and you won't be as likely to overeat.

Write in a Journal

Getting your thoughts and experiences down on paper can help in reducing stress. Writing often untangles your thoughts and feelings and gives you insight into why you do what you do.

You can also journal what you eat every day, helping to keep yourself accountable. You can commit your goals to paper, which will make you more conscious of what you want to accomplish and where you're headed.

Consider These Basic Guidelines to Manage Stress

If we tend to be emotional eaters in times of stress, we resort to food. Be aware of these potential stressors: personal loss, financial problems, job changes (even good ones), major illness or injury, retirement, etc. If you find you're facing any of these or other stressors, try the following:

- See your doctor to help treat physical or psychological symptoms caused by stress and to give you the okay on exercise. Exercise helps to reduce stress, increases your endorphins, and calms you down. See Chapter 16 on exercise.

- Eat properly and drink lots of water. Reduce your intake of sugar, which gives you a brief energy boost, followed by a crash, and will deplete your resources for handling stress. Increase your B-Complex and C vitamins, which are depleted during stress. Limit alcohol, as this disrupts your sleep cycle. Cut down on smoking (if you smoke), as nicotine is a stimulant that produces stress.

- Make sleep a priority! Getting 7-9 hours is best. It helps to handle stress if we have had enough sleep. See Chapter 15 on sleep.

- Take time out to disengage. Reading fiction has been shown to be better than walking (we still need to exercise) to reduce stress. When we read, our minds go into a "trance-like" state, almost like meditation, and we get the same benefits as deep relaxation. If we read regularly, we sleep better, lower our stress, and decrease the chance of depression. Research out of the University of Sussex indicates that reading fiction is more effective in reducing stress than taking a walk or listening to music.[3]

- Prioritize your work.

- Clearly communicate your wants and needs.

Stress Tips

Other Actions to Consider

- Talk to a counselor about things you don't talk to a friend about. It helps.

- Surround yourself with more people who are positive and begin to weed out those who aren't. Don't let others bring you down. Move on with your life.

- Play with a pet.

- Get a coloring book! I'm not kidding. It can be very relaxing.

- Create the habit of being thankful.

- Volunteer.

- Get involved with people, whether through sports, church, or social groups.

- Make sure your expectations are realistic.

- At Christmas time, don't overspend and have credit card debt you can't pay in January.

- Don't procrastinate!

- Smile!
- Be good to yourself with compliments and rewards for reaching goals.
- Stop personalizing! It's not always about you.
- Keep your house picked up. Get rid of what you don't need or love.
- Take time for what you're passionate about.

Go to page 43 in your journal and list what stress management tools you will use.

An important part of dealing with stress is letting go. Let me end this chapter with information a client gave me at work. There's no reference to an author. I wish I could give credit because it's excellent! Enjoy!

To "Let Go" Takes Love

To "let go" does not mean to stop caring; it means I can't do it for someone else.

To "let go" is not to cut myself off; it is the realization I can't control another.

To "let go" is not to enable, but to allow learning from natural consequences.

To "let go" is to admit powerlessness, which means the outcome is not in my hands.

To "let go" is not to try to change or blame another; it is to make the most of myself.

To "let go" is not to care for, but to care about.

To "let go" is not to fix, but to be supportive.

To "let go" is not to judge, but to allow another to be a human being.

To "let go" is not to be in the middle arranging all the outcomes, but to allow others to affect their own destinies.

To "let go" is not to be protective; it is to permit another to face reality.

To "let go" is not to deny, but to accept.

To "let go" is not to nag, scold, or argue, but instead to search out my own shortcomings and to correct them.

To "let go" is not to adjust everything to my desires but to take each day as it comes, and to cherish myself in it.

To "let go" is not to criticize and regulate anybody, but to try to become what I dream I can be.

To "let go" is not regretting the past, but to grow and to live for the future.

To "let go" is to fear less and to love more.

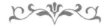

Chapter 15:
Sleep, Glorious Sleep!

"It is in vain that you rise up early and go late to rest, eating the bread of anxious toil; for he gives to his beloved sleep."
—Psalms 127:2 (English Standard Version)

In the movie "Oliver Twist," the characters cry out, "Food, glorious food!"[1] With our busy schedules and lack of sleep, we should cry out, "Sleep, glorious sleep!" Sleep is *so* important to our well-being, and yet we don't give it its proper due. We pack in extra work, maximizing every bit of our waking day and on into the night, being as productive as we can, yet at what cost? Are we really as productive as we think we are? And what is the cost to our battles with our weight?

A few years ago, *The New York Times,* which is notorious for denying health claims, supported claims made by researchers that a lack of sleep increases your weight. Sleep and weight loss/weight maintenance go hand in hand. This correlates with studies that show your appetite hormones are thrown out of whack. Ghrelin is the hormone that causes you to be hungry, and it increases with lack of sleep. Less sleep, more hunger. Leptin, on the other hand, lets us know when we're full, and this hormone decreases with lack of sleep.

With less sleep, we continue eating because we don't know when we're full.

In a study done in 2005 with 8,000 adults, the National Health and Nutrition Examination Survey found that less than seven hours of sleep a night correlated with a greater risk of weight gain and obesity. The risk continued to rise for every hour of lost sleep under seven hours. In a further study, the *American Journal of Clinical Nutrition* reported on a study where men slept one night for eight hours and the next night they slept for four hours. On the day after the short night, the men ate 500 more calories (about a 22% increase). Over the course of a week, that would add up to a one-pound weight gain.[2] In a year's time, you could pack on 52 pounds by not getting enough sleep each night.

Another study out of the University of Chicago found that both men and women ate more calories in snack and junk food after getting 5.5 hours of sleep as opposed to 8.5 hours of sleep at night.

According to Dr. Susan Peirce Thompson, rats deprived of leptin will continue to eat, appearing to become three to four times the size of normal rats; the only exercise they get is when the food dish is moved from them, and they follow it to continue eating.[3] Very interesting! This is something we can fix! If you're having problems with sleep, check with your doctor; you may be a candidate for a sleep evaluation.

Other than helping us to manage our weight, why is sleep important? "Let me count the ways." It gives us more energy and helps in managing our stress levels as well as improving our overall well-being and mood. When we sleep, we restore and recharge our bodies and increase our ability to manage our willpower. If we skimp on sleep (7-8 hours is recommended, and some authorities recommend between 7.5 and 9.5 hours to not be sleep deprived), it affects every system in our bodies. It also helps with memory, learning, and academic performance. When we see all the reasons to get more sleep, it can increase our motivation to make it a priority. Here are some other ways it affects us. Let's start with weight loss.

Benefits of Sleep

1. It helps in weight maintenance.

Although sleep doesn't cause us to lose weight, it can help us by not adding extra pounds as well as helping us to maintain healthy eating habits. We have already discussed the impact of sleep on ghrelin and leptin. According to Dr. Jen Ashton on a "Good Morning America" segment, when we're sleep deprived, our body thinks something is wrong and consumes lean muscle instead of body fat.[4] That is *not* what we want! We want to have lean muscle mass to help burn calories, and we want our bodies to burn the fat, not the other way around.

When we're more fatigued from lack of a good night's rest, we're more prone to give in to junk food cravings, as was noted in the studies above. On a personal note, while writing this book, one night I woke up every hour but was able to go back to sleep. Nevertheless, I was tired. The next day was NOT a good day! I had no willpower and gave in to eating much more than I should have, all because of a lack of a good night's rest.

2. Getting good sleep helps with managing our insulin's effectiveness.

Dr. Jen Ashton also reported that when a study was done at the Sutter Health CPMC Hospital (Pacific Campus) and the subjects had eight hours of sleep, their bodies were able to convert glucose as it should; it was only up about 6%, which is well within the body's ability to process it with insulin. When the subjects were sleep-deprived, even for one night, insulin lost its efficiency by 21%. This can lead to an increased risk for diabetes and metabolic disorders.

3. Getting enough sleep keeps your heart healthy.

If we are sleep-deprived, it places an extra toll on our hearts, which can lead to heart health problems, including high blood pressure and heart attacks. When we don't get regular good sleep, we subject our bodies to higher levels of stress hormones, such as cortisol. With the added stress from these hormones, your heart compensates and has to work harder and doesn't get to restore itself, according to Dr. Shalini Paruthi, M.D., a sleep specialist and spokesperson for the American Academy of Sleep Medicine.[5] With added stress, we tend to "comfort eat" all the wrong foods.

4. It reduces your risk of being in a car crash.

Did you know that driving while being sleep-deprived is as dangerous as driving drunk? Yes. You heard me correctly. It's as dangerous as driving drunk. When you're sleep-deprived, your reaction time is slowed, and your ability to focus is compromised. This is not even considering dozing off behind the wheel for even a few seconds. Research indicates you're twice as likely to be in a car accident on 6 to 7 hours of sleep on a regular basis than are those people who get a regular 8 hours of sleep, according to a study from the AAA Foundation for Traffic Safety. If you get less than 5 hours of sleep regularly, your chances of a car crash quadruples.[5] Does this make you want to go to bed earlier?

5. Your immune system is improved by sleep.

When you don't get enough sleep, inflammation in your body is increased. This increases the risk of cardiovascular disease, cancer, major depression, and irritability. If you want to be healthier and keep from being off work with colds and the flu, make sleep a priority and a regular habit to keep your immune system in tip-top shape. If you're getting a vaccine, regular sleep makes it more effective, according to Dr. Paruthi. If you have sleep issues, you don't develop the same antibody protection as people who are well rested.[5]

6. Sleep improves your sex life.

Getting quality sleep keeps testosterone levels high and helps to prevent erectile dysfunction. For men, less than six hours of sleep a night will lower testosterone levels. For both men and women, it insures not being too tired to keep the intimacy alive.[5]

7. Sleep helps prevent headaches.

If you're prone to getting headaches from stress, regular sleep will decrease your stress levels and increase your ability to handle the stress that does come your way. According to Dr. Paruthi, being deprived of sleep indirectly plays a role in your headaches and decreases your ability to cope with stress and anxiety, which can trigger your headache. It can also lead to stress eating.[5]

8. Sleep helps with top performance at the gym.

When you get good quality sleep, your speed, eye-hand coordination, reaction time and muscle recovery are much better than if you work out being sleep deprived. It doesn't take much of not getting enough sleep to throw off your workout. In 2013, a study was done and reported in the *Journal of Strength and Conditioning Research,* that with sleep deprivation, there was a decrease in muscle strength and power the next day.[5] If you're going to put the blood, sweat, and tears into your workout at the gym, it makes sense to maximize your efforts by getting enough sleep.

9. Good sleep increases positive relationships.

When you don't get enough good-quality sleep, you're more cranky and irritable and have less empathy for others. As a parent, sleep helps you to be more consistent with discipline guidelines given to your children. It also gives you the strength to set boundaries with others and end toxic relationships, if needed. Good sleep is a protection against mindless, emotional eating from frustrations with others and gives you the willpower to choose better.

10. Getting regular good REM sleep helps to maintain good mental health.

When we get good sleep, we wake up refreshed and positive about the day ahead. We're less likely to be stressed and irritable and more able to cope with whatever challenges we may face.

I don't know if you remember the Public Service Announcement (PSA) in the 1980s, comparing a fried egg to your brain on drugs. So is your brain on sleep deprivation. If you're not sleeping, you're not dreaming. Good restful sleep helps us with concentration and better cognitive functioning, whereas even one sleepless night leaves us feeling "fuzzyheaded, scattered, and unfocused the next day," according to Dr. Paruthi. Your memory recall is not as sharp, and you function much more slowly than you would if you had enough sleep. This can put your job at risk with increased mistakes, which you're less likely to recognize and correct.[5]

Studies have been done on the effect of REM sleep deprival (dream deprival) but still being allowed to go back to sleep. As Harold Sampson, Ph.D. states in, "Psychological Effects of Deprivation of Dreaming Sleep," those involved in the study reported an increase in appetite and cravings, irritability, and difficulty in concentrating and focusing. Depersonalization, memory problems (forgetting appointments), motor coordination, intense hunger, and "formed hallucinations" with a distorted sense of reality during deprivation, were also noted.[6]

Every subject in the study also noted an increase in appetite, feeling hungry all the time. After going out for a meal, one college student felt intensely hungry just one hour later. The next day, he continued to experience "intense hunger, ate six times today."[6]

Irritability was an expected outcome in the study, but what stood out was the intensity of the reaction, appearing to be regressive in childish behavior. Paranoid themes also were present. Others were confused and illogical in their thought processes.[6]

In your journal on page 45, consider the benefits of sleep. Which ones stood out to you? How much sleep do you get each night? Is it enough? If not, what can you do to get more sleep?

Concluding Remarks

Getting more sleep has many benefits to our health and well-being and success in losing weight and weight control. That's one area we can easily make a priority. Getting good sleep will lead to an abundance of return on our investment!

I know your struggles with sleep. While growing up, my mother engaged me in mother-daughter time watching old movies late into the night and the wee early morning hours. I became a "night owl." I went off to college, taking my "night owl" habits with me, wanting to excel in school. Since our society values productivity, it was easy to use those wee hours to squeeze in as much work as possible. You may say, "Yes, but I have children waking me up during the night." That comes with parenting. What about taking a nap when they do, instead of folding laundry? You will be much more productive when you're rested, and it will help your weight-loss efforts.

Getting good sleep will lead to an abundance of return on our investment!

The good news is I'm a recovered "night owl," and you can be, too. When you look at the tradeoff of staying up to get that "one more thing" done with being so unproductive the next day, you will begin to value sleep. Remember the Stanford Marshmallow Experiment? It can work for sleep, too—instant gratification versus long-term benefit. Just like anything else, it will be tempting to stay up, but you must *choose* each night to go to bed (set a timer as a reminder to begin to get ready, if you need to), being confident that you will have a better day tomorrow. It's time to reclaim getting a good night's sleep!

Tips to Improve Sleep

Your Personal Habits

- Prioritizing sleep is a must! Make going to bed at a regular time to get eight hours of sleep each night a daily habit. Avoid long naps in the day, which will affect your sleep routines. Also, get up at the same time every morning (even weekends) to ensure you will be ready to sleep at your regular bedtime.

- Monitor not eating after dinner. Avoid heavy, spicy, or sugary food 4-6 hours before bed. Don't eat after 3 hours before bed, if at all possible. Your body needs time to digest the food before sleeping so your body isn't working all night, causing a bad night's sleep, leaving you tired the next day. Try brushing and flossing your teeth to prevent having a later snack. When mice had a fasting period eating the same calories as those who snacked around the clock, the mice with a controlled time to eat stayed lean whereas the other mice became obese with round-the-clock eating (same calories).

- If you're hungry a couple of hours before bed, try a light snack of a few almonds, a banana, a glass of skim milk, or some oatmeal. Watch portion sizes.

- Avoid caffeine (coffee, tea, cola, chocolate), especially in the afternoon, so it will be out of your system by bedtime. If you're still having trouble, try backing it up to the morning.

- Avoid smoking and alcohol before bed. It may cause withdrawals, waking you up and giving you poor quality sleep.

- Get regular exposure to daylight for at least 20 minutes a day, especially gazing at the sunrise or sunset. This helps to regulate specific chemicals and hormones, such as melatonin, which are important for sleep, mood, and aging.

- Get regular exercise, which can help you sleep better, but don't work out vigorously before bed (at least a few hours before to give you time to wind down). It increases your cortisol levels and gets you ready to be productive. Have you ever gone for a jog on your lunch break and come back refreshed for the afternoon instead of having that mid-afternoon slump?

- Our lives are bombarded with stimuli: late dinners (the worst thing for weight loss—you pack on the pounds and you don't get restful sleep because your body is working to digest the food instead of bringing restorative sleep), answering emails, checking social media, surfing the web, working, or watching TV before crashing into bed. The blue light from electronic gadgets (computers and especially cell phones) can slow down the production of melatonin, which can help you sleep.

Your Environment for Sleep

- Make sure you have a comfortable mattress. Try using lavender on your sheets and pillows.

- Use your bed for sleep and/or romance only. This signals your body for sleep. No TV in bed. It keeps your mind wired for activity.

- Make the environment aesthetically pleasing with calm colors, getting rid of clutter and distractions.

- Make the room completely dark. Use an eye mask and ear plugs, if needed.

- Turn on a small fan or white noise machine to lull you to sleep to mask any sudden noise that might wake you.

Getting Ready For Bed

- Prepare for sleep by having bedtime rituals, such as reading, listening to music, practicing relaxation techniques, such as yoga or deep breathing to reduce muscle tension or anxiety. Even laughing can put you in a better mood for sleep. It's a time to wind down to physically and psychologically prepare for bed and going to sleep.

- Some people like to make their To Do Lists for the next day. If you can't fall asleep, try reading until you begin to feel sleepy or try deep breathing exercises. Have a notebook by the side of the bed to write down anything that is bothering you. Getting things out onto paper causes you to not have to hold onto it while trying to sleep, giving you more restful sleep.

- Take a hot bath before bed. Raising your body temperature induces sleep. Relaxing in a hot tub relaxes your muscles and reduces tension. If you add equal portions of Epsom salt and baking soda (one half cup to one cup each), you will benefit from the magnesium being absorbed through your skin and the baking soda has alkaline to balance the effects. Both help with sleep.

- You might consider trying meditation or a guided imagery CD to help you relax while going to sleep. You may find rainfall or ocean sounds relaxing by using electronic devices or CDs.

- Stretch before bed or have your spouse or partner massage you.

Other Factors to Talk to Your Doctor About

- Avoid medications that interfere with sleep. You don't want to become dependent on them and experience the drowsy effects that carry over into the next day. Watch out for headache medications that contain caffeine, and if you're on stimulant medication for ADHD, make sure it will be out of your system before bed. Check with your doctor to see if any medications you take can cause you to have a hard time going to sleep.

- Try using herbal therapies one hour before bed. Valerian root extract (500 mg) is an effective herbal sleep aid. You can also take 200-400 mg of magnesium, which relaxes your muscles and nervous system. You can get help with this from your local health and vitamin store. Always check with your doctor before taking supplements, as there may be an adverse impact on your current health condition and medications you're taking.[7]

- If sleep is a continuing problem after using these techniques, it never hurts to be checked out by your doctor for problems that could interfere with sleep, such as food sensitivities, thyroid problems, menopause, fibromyalgia, chronic fatigue syndrome, heavy metal toxicity, not to mention stress and depression. While you're with your doctor, consider being screened for a sleep disorder, such as sleep apnea.

In the next chapter on exercise, we will come full circle with exercise, which helps in the areas of weight loss, stress reduction, and better sleeping. Actually, they're all intertwined, affecting each other. Better sleep makes it easier to lose weight, reduces stress, and gives you more energy to exercise. Managing stress helps with sleeping and our eating habits, and exercise helps to manage our stress, going to sleep, giving us better moods, which helps in decreasing the desire to "comfort eat." Let's continue reading ...

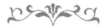

Chapter 16:
Exercise—It Really ISN'T the "E" Word

*"Take care of your body. It's the only place you
have to live."*—Jim Rohn

When it comes to exercise, there are two camps of people—those who love it and the endorphins it produces, and those who hate it, who *really* hate it. In either case, exercise is an integral part of our well-being.

**Before beginning any exercise program, check with
your doctor for any underlying conditions that
would need to be monitored or accommodated.**

You're probably well aware of exercise as being a part of any weight-loss or weight-management program. Our weight is dependent on the number of calories taken in minus the calories expended, which equals weight loss or weight gain. Exercise increases our metabolism, which aids in calories being burned at a higher rate, even when we're not engaged in exercise.

Many people don't like to exercise; getting into a routine of regular exercise helps. Pick an exercise you're more likely to participate in and link it to something you want to do afterward; you look forward to the reward for actually getting it done.

Let's look at an example. You know you need to exercise. The cue is feeling tired or having gained some weight and wanting to take it off. The reward is more energy, a sense of well-being, and losing some weight.

What will the routine be? You want to run in the morning. You lay out your running clothes and shoes by your bed the night before. When you wake up, you put on your running attire and shoes, which signals you to get ready for your run. When you are finished, you are ready to begin your day with more energy and a refreshed perspective.

Exercise ... aids in calories being burned at a higher rate, even when we're not engaged in exercise.

If you're not a morning person, but you know you won't exercise once the day gets started, you can begin slowly by walking, then speed walking, then jogging. If you can find an exercise buddy, accountability helps.

If you're a stay-at-home mom or have flexibility in your day, you can use the above example for the how-to. You're free to exercise any time in the day. It's easy to put it off until it doesn't happen. Think about linking exercise to another activity in your day. Example: exercise, and then make breakfast or lunch or dinner. You can link exercise before picking up children from school or right after dropping them off.

What Types of Exercises Should I Do?

Our bodies are meant to move and get exercise. A combination of cardiovascular exercise and strength training will yield numerous health benefits in a relatively short time (a few weeks).

When determining what exercises to include in your routine, it depends on what your goals are. It would be ideal to include all three types—aerobic exercise, resistance training, and core exercises.[1]

Aerobic Exercise

Aerobic or cardiovascular exercise gets your heart pumping, and aerobic means to exercise "with oxygen." You want to get your heart rate between 65%-85% of your maximum heart rate. Examples of aerobic exercise include jogging, cycling, swimming, power walking, boxing, rowing, dancing, tennis, basketball, soccer, and jumping rope, to name a few.

Along with aerobic exercise, you can vary it by using interval training, which includes alternating high intensity exercise with periods of lower intensity exercise.

Goals of an Aerobic Exercise Program[2]

- It should be aerobic, using large muscles for a sustained amount of time.

- It should be done for 30-60 minutes, three to five times per week.

- It should meet your cardiovascular goals set for you by either your doctor or a trainer at the gym.

- It should be something you will enjoy doing.

The benefits of aerobic exercise within your target heart rate are:

- reduced body fat
- improvement in heart and lung function, decreasing your chances of developing heart disease
- lower blood pressure and resting pulse
- lowering insulin resistance
- producing endorphins, which are natural chemicals that help with reducing pain and enhancing mood for your well-being

Resistance Exercise

Resistance exercise entails exactly what it implies—resistance with use of weights (dumbbells or barbells), resistance bands, medicine balls, or your own body weight. Benefits include:

- increased metabolism as you increase muscle
- better posture
- improved muscular strength and agility
- better tendon and ligament strength

Core Stability Exercises

Core stability exercises strengthen your muscles around your lumbar spine and pelvis area. They stabilize your trunk region, which then provides a strong base for all movement. If you're moving correctly, your movement should come from your core.

Why Do I Need to Exercise and What are the Health Benefits?

If you can see health benefits to exercise, you will find many reasons and motivation to exercise! Here they are:

Physical Benefits of Exercise

1. Exercise helps to control your weight.

Exercise keeps us from excess weight gain (if we watch what we eat); it helps us to maintain our weight loss, once we have achieved our goals. Exercising burns calories and increases our metabolism to burn more calories. You don't need a gym membership to exercise (see the examples above). The more intense your workout is, the more calories you burn. You can also burn calories by taking the stairs instead of the elevator and by parking further away in the parking lot to get in a few more minutes of walking. You can probably think of other examples as well.

It doesn't take long when you start exercising for your metabolism to be increased. When your heart rate goes up and your circulation increases, your brain responds and produces neurochemicals that boost your mood and your metabolism, according to Rebecca Jaffe, M.D., a family doctor who is a member of the Board of Directors for the American Academy of Family Physicians. Your increased metabolism can last from a few hours to a few days, but for continued increased metabolism, you have to continue to exercise regularly to maintain the benefit.[3]

2. It will lower your blood pressure.

Sara Schwartz cites several other benefits to exercise from various researchers. According to Randi S. Lite, Associate Professor of Practice and Director of the Exercise Science Program at Simmons College, there is a reduction in resting blood pressure for 24-48 hours after moderate cardiovascular exercise. As we get older, our blood vessels stiffen, which increases blood pressure. Dr. Rani Whitfield, a family doctor and American Heart Association spokesperson, tells us our bodies release hormones during exercise that make our blood vessels more compliant (to yield elastically when a force is applied) or more flexible. This result is similar to what blood pressure medications do, according to Dr. Whitfield. If we can get the same result with exercise before needing medication, why not give it a try? Along with decreasing your risk for heart disease, you can also prevent or manage other health problems, such as stroke, metabolic syndrome, diabetes, depression, some cancers, arthritis, and falls.

3. It will regulate your blood sugar.

When we exercise, we use the glucose in our bodies (blood sugar for fuel), and exercising improves our bodies' use of insulin (the hormone that regulates our blood sugar), according to Dr. Whitfield. The good news is that when a person becomes fit, their doctor can make adjustments to their medications for diabetes.

4. You will be able to lift more weight with stronger muscles.

After a few weeks of weight training and exercise, your muscles will actually "become smarter and more efficient," according to Randi Lite. You will be able to lift more weight with less effort, and you may notice you can now bound up the stairs instead of dragging yourself one step at a time. Your nervous system is reprogramming muscle fiber used to lift weight and move your body.

5. You will have less arthritis pain.

According to Dr. Jaffe, you can relieve arthritis pain in your joints in as little as two weeks. When you have arthritis, the shock-absorbing cartilage between bones is weakened. When you strengthen the muscles around the knees and shoulders, it takes the stress off the joint. You may say, "I'm in too much pain to exercise." Try exercising in a pool 30 minutes three times a week for two weeks and see the results.

6. It can help control addictions.

When people use harmful substances and participate in activities that can be negatively addicting, the dopamine (the "reward chemical") that is released delivers different forms of pleasure. In the process, some people become addicted to the dopamine and the substance causing its release. Exercise can help. Short exercise sessions can distract users, and they can learn to handle cravings in the short term. Working out when sober helps to regulate sleep patterns, so the alcoholic doesn't have to rely on alcohol to fall asleep.

Studies have shown exercise can help curb alcohol dependency by increasing mood, decreasing depressive symptoms, and providing improved coping behaviors. For nicotine cravings and withdrawal, symptoms decreased during exercise and results lasted for about 50 minutes, enough time to get involved in another activity.

7. You will feel much better.

According to Janelle W. Coughlin, Ph.D., Assistant Professor at the Johns Hopkins School of Medicine, Department of Psychiatry and Behavioral Health, studies have shown that almost all exercise improves depression and increases self-esteem. Patients often report better sleep and feeling more energetic, more confident and more motivated shortly after increasing exercise in the first few weeks. Exercise increases blood flow to the brain. Our bodies are more able to handle stress. When we exercise, we produce more endorphins and feel better emotionally. We get a boost with social interaction (if exercising with others), handle distractions better, and improve our self-confidence with the knowledge of improving our health.

Leoni Epiphaniou is a psychotherapist in the Boston area. She helps clients learn to deal with stress, anxiety, trauma, depression, and other problems. On the side, she's a Zumba instructor and believes that exercise, especially dance, helps you to let go and achieve healing that's difficult with only talk therapy. She believes that learning a new dance routine and "being in the moment" helps to interrupt negative thoughts.

Benefits of Zumba include:

- It's easy to do and can be a lot of fun. It helps you to have a more optimistic posture, which helps with brighter thoughts and feelings.

- You have a social connection with camaraderie with the others in the group. Zumba classes promote social interaction, which can lead to increased happiness and confidence.

- It helps with mindfulness. When you focus on the present moment to feel the beat and learn a routine, you lose yourself in moving and dancing. You don't focus on your anxiety about your past or future. You're in the here-and-now, and it helps to break negative thought patterns, along with cultivating relaxation, being positive and aware, which increases optimum functioning with increased energy and health.[5]

8. Other benefits with 30 minutes of exercise three days a week include:

- A stronger immune system
- More energy
- Less stiffness
- Decreased cholesterol levels
- Decreased risk of falling due to improved balance and coordination

Emotional Benefits of Exercise

Exercise will give you emotional benefits besides helping with calories being burned and health improvements. Check these out:[6]

1. It will reduce stress.

Exercising is one of the most common ways to reduce stress, and it increases the concentration of norepinephrine, a chemical that helps us to respond to stress. An added benefit is that it increases our ability to deal with existing mental tensions.

2. It increases your "happy" chemicals.

When you exercise, you increase your endorphins, which bring on feelings of happiness and sometimes euphoria. Studies have shown the efficacy of exercise in reducing depressive symptoms. In some cases, it has been shown to be as effective as antidepressants. Just 30 minutes three times a week can boost your overall mood.

3. It will improve your self-confidence.

Even if you're overweight, exercising to improve your overall fitness can improve your self-esteem and give you a more positive self-image. Exercise gives you a sense of overall well-being and increases your perception of yourself.

4. Consider exercising in the great outdoors.

This boosts your self-esteem even more. Find an activity you enjoy, such as hiking, rock climbing, jogging, etc. The vitamin D from the sun protects against multiple diseases and conditions, such as osteoporosis, cancer, type 1 diabetes, and multiple sclerosis, and the serotonin lessens your chances of experiencing symptoms of depression.

5. It can alleviate anxiety.

People with anxiety disorders calm down after jogging for 20-30 minutes. If you go to the gym and use the treadmill for moderate-to-high aerobics, the use of interval training reduces being sensitive to anxiety. It's not just for burning extra calories!

6. It increases relaxation.

Moderate exercise helps with insomnia. When you work out about 5 to 6 hours before bed, your body temperature is raised, and when it drops back down, it signals the body for sleep.

Intellectual Benefits of Exercise

1. It helps cognitive decline.

As we get older, our brains actually begin to shrink. Exercise and healthy eating help protect the brain from cognitive decline, especially between the ages of 25 and 45. It increases the chemicals in the brain that support and prevent the degeneration of the hippocampus, which is the center for memory and learning.

2. It boosts your brain power.

We now know that cardiovascular exercise creates new brain cells, a process known as neurogenesis. It also increases overall brain performance, including decision-making, higher thought processing, and learning.

3. It sharpens your memory.

If you want to boost your memory and ability to learn new things, you need to engage in regular physical activity. When you are sweaty from exercise, there's an increased production of cells in your hippocampus, which is responsible for memory and learning. That's why exercise for children is important because their brains are continuing to develop.

4. You get more done.

If you take regular time for exercise, you will be more productive and have more energy than those who are sedentary. Due to circadian rhythms, some experts advocate midday as the best time for exercise. Others advocate mornings to rev up your metabolism, but it is more important to work with your schedule to be consistent to get in a minimum of 30 minutes three to five times a week.

5. It gives you time for creativity.

If you want to increase your creativity, try tapping into it after you've worked out. The benefits should last for a few hours, and you may have a breakthrough in a task or project where you were otherwise stuck.

6. You can be an inspiration for others.

When you exercise with a buddy, you can inspire each other to push your limits and perform at a higher rate as a result. The accountability is good for socialization and consistency for both of you.

Before leaving this chapter, assess your exercise habits. Go to page 47 in your journal to list the reasons that are important to you to exercise. What are they? If you're not exercising, find a time and exercise plan that will work in your schedule. When and what will it be?

In Summary

Exercise helps with weight loss by increasing our metabolism and burning calories. It has many other benefits, including physical, emotional, and intellectual benefits. When I'm not feeling very motivated to exercise, it helps to think beyond just my weight-loss efforts and to look at all the wonderful benefits there are to exercising, and that is usually what does the trick! It does a body good!

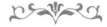

THE PROMISE

The Promise

"Hope deferred makes the heart sick, but a
longing fulfilled is a tree of life."
—Proverbs 13:12 (New International Version)

After you have lost your weight, you will be glad you did! It
might be easy to think, "I'm free now!" and be a little more
lax on what and how much you eat. Don't! You have worked
too hard. Don't go back to your old ways. Embrace your new
lifestyle and allow your new body image to be congruent with
who you want to be. Enjoy the new you!

You may have already experienced "yo-yo" dieting in the
past. Did you embrace a new image of yourself, or did you go
back to your old eating habits from your internalized image
of being a "fat" person? Once you have lost the weight, you
don't want to have to do it again and again. How painful and
frustrating is that!

You have probably heard the idea that weight management
involves a lifestyle change. Usually it refers to changing what
and how you eat. I would like to propose the idea that a
lifestyle change includes not only healthy eating but also
continuing to implement all the principles in this book that
helped you to lose the weight in the first place. Having lost
the weight isn't a free pass to return to eating the way you

did that caused you to become overweight in the first place. Just remember, "Do you want the 'one marshmallow' of instant gratification or 'two marshmallows' of long-term reward?" You can claim what is rightfully yours—a life where you can be free, confident, and happy without weight issues consuming your thoughts all the time.

You have to see yourself with this new body image day after day. You have to embrace the new you! Do you remember reading that fat people tend to gain weight? You have to let your mind catch up with your body so that you see yourself as trim and slim. Then you will take action to be consistent with how you see yourself *now*.

> *You have to let your mind catch up with your body so that you see yourself as trim and slim.*

If you want a life free of yo-yo dieting or gaining the weight back and becoming complacent about it, you have to stop the excuses, watch out for sabotaging behaviors by yourself and others, stop rationalizing by giving yourself permission to eat what you know you shouldn't, watch for triggers, change habits, manage stress, get sleep, and exercise.

This may seem overwhelming, but take one area (e.g., sleep) and work on it until it becomes automatic. Then you can take the next area, and so on. Hopefully, you're already implementing much of this from shedding those pounds. Great job!

You are on your way to being more confident, having more energy, being free from obsession about your weight, and being much happier! This is the life you have worked so hard for. Now go live it!

ADDENDUM

Basic Guidelines on Weight Loss

1. Journal everything you're eating. Include what you eat, when you eat it, how you're feeling at the time you're eating. If you find you're an emotional eater, try making a list of things you can do instead of eating. If you're still having trouble, consider talking to a counselor for help to learn how to manage your emotions.

2. Once your eating plan is in place, make exercise a priority. Don't forget the importance of sleep and managing your stress. Exercise, sleep, and stress management go hand-in-hand and affect each other.

3. Get support from friends and family. Let them know what you're trying to do and enlist their help. Educate them on how not to sabotage your efforts.

4. Find an accountability partner. There's nothing like accountability! If we know that we will have to report our progress at the end of the week, it motivates us to stay the course. By setting a goal for the week, you have a target to guide your behaviors. An accountability partner can encourage you when you're down, and you can do the same for him/her.

5. Make decisions based on your core values and goals. Don't let others persuade you otherwise. They don't go home with you, and they don't live your life.

6. Keep a visual picture of your new self in the forefront of your thinking. Start your day with visualizing the new you.

Other Guidelines to Consider

The indulgences for special occasions don't wreak havoc with our weight loss efforts, but, rather our everyday habits do, and we may not even be aware of them. Here are some bad habits from the editors of *Eat This, Not That.*[1]

1. You eat "low-fat."

When a food is marketed as "low-fat," the fats have been replaced by carbohydrates that don't give energy; they digest quickly, and they result in hunger in a short time. Some fat in your meal causes you to feel fuller longer and causes you to be less likely to snack later. See Tip #15.

2. You ignore nutritional advice.

If you're interested in weight loss or weight management, you need to be informed about your habits that can help you lose or maintain your weight. The good news is you have already begun by reading this book to make these changes.

3. You sleep too little or too much. Please see the tips given in Chapter 15 on sleep.

4. You eat free restaurant food, such as chips and salsa and bread.

This may be "free" in dollars, but it definitely isn't free when your clothes don't fit anymore or the number on the scale goes up. You have to budget your calories just as you budget your money.

5. You drink soda, even diet soda.

Giving up 150 calories from soda helps in cutting calories. You won't feel that much hungrier, and you can use those calories for "real" food that will fill you up and nourish your body. You may wonder about diet soda since it has no calories. The problem with diet sodas is that the artificial sweetener causes you to want to eat more, so you do without even realizing it; hence, you're prone to gain weight from it. It also causes an increase in your insulin levels, which then holds onto extra fat. This definitely defeats the purpose of a diet soda.

Drink water instead. See Tip #20.

6. You skip meals.

Skipping meals reduces your metabolism because your body is responding to a "famine." This sets you up to overeat or snack on comfort food later in the day because you're hungry.

7. You eat too quickly.

When you eat too quickly, you eat a lot more than if you ate more slowly. It takes about 20 minutes for you to feel full. By that time, you have packed in a lot more food than if you had slowed down. Try chewing your food 100 times, putting your fork down in between bites, or participate in the conversation at mealtime.

8. You watch too much TV.

Sitting too much is the "new smoking." Our bodies are meant for movement. If you must watch, try ironing, washing dishes, or folding laundry while listening. If you don't want to miss your favorite drama, record it, and fast forward through the commercials to be sitting less. If you leave the commercials on, get up to do something while waiting for the program to return. How about doing some jumping jacks or jump rope?

9. You order the combo meal.

Do you really need all that food? What about healthier choices?

10. You face the buffet.

If you're serious about losing weight, avoid this at all cost. If you must go to a buffet for work or with friends, make healthy choices and go through the line once. You'll be glad you did.

11. You drink out of plastic.

We don't know the effect of all the chemicals in our plastics, so it's better to drink from glass (try a mason jar). Try adding any combination of grapefruit, mint, oranges, limes, lemons, cucumbers, strawberries, blueberries for a refreshing cooler.

12. You don't let off steam.

Take time to relax and stretch. See tips for stress reduction in Chapter 14 on stress.

13. You don't moderate your diet.

Plan what you will eat. Make a list of what you will need when you go to the grocery store. When your week begins, plan your evening meals and what you will take to work for lunch. It really won't take that much longer, and you will be glad you did.

14. You don't go for a physical.

Get a good physical to rule out medical causes for weight problems. While you're seeing the doctor, ask for a nutritional consultation and recommendations for exercise.

15. You avoid all fats.

We need some fats to feel full longer. Don't be afraid of adding avocados and olive oil to your meals. All in moderation, of course.

16. You don't ask how it's cooked.

By the very nature of eating out, you will consume many more calories, fats, sodium, and MSG than if you ate at home. You can choose fish, poultry, or meat that's grilled or broiled without the butter sauce. High levels of sodium raise our blood pressure and our water retention. Don't be afraid to ask. It's your body you're watching out for.

17. You ignore sodium counts.

18. You eat off large plates.

Try a smaller size plate (9" plate), eat more slowly, and see that you didn't really miss the larger portions. Don't go back for seconds, which defeats the purpose. Portion control is important!

19. You serve from the table.

This makes the food readily available for seconds and thirds. Out of sight, out of mind.

20. You don't drink enough water.

Sometimes, we find ourselves eating when we're really dehydrated without even realizing it. Drinking water helps to keep us hydrated, and we avoid a multitude of physical symptoms. It also helps in digestion and burning of calories.

21. You hang out with unhealthy friends.

If your friends have different health and fitness values than you do, it may be time to make some friends who can support you in your weight-loss goals or rally them to join you in making changes.

22. You use a scale.

There has been some controversy on this one. Some say to weigh once a week to not be obsessed with your weight and to focus on healthy eating. Others weigh themselves daily to have an accountability check and to remind themselves to stay on track.

23. You drink alcohol and fruit juices.

Fruit juices wallop concentrated calories and a sugar spike whereas eating the fruit itself packs in more nutrients and fiber and is easier on your system. Alcohol has empty calories, increases appetite, slows down your metabolism, and decreases your willpower, not to mention a hangover the next day.

24. You don't drink the right tea.

Here's a list of five teas that will help you in weight loss:

Green tea—boosts your metabolism.

Oolong tea—"melts" calories.

Mint tea—decreases cravings.

White tea—helps to block fat.

Rooibos tea—decreases hunger.

Here are some other things to consider:

1. Know how many calories you need to eat and then subtract 500 calories to lose a pound a week.

2. Eat more of your meals at home. You can control how it's prepared and save a few hundred calories, not to mention dollars. If you must eat out, decide how much you want to eat, and then save the rest to go home in a "doggie bag" for lunch the next day.

3. Eat a variety of food. This brings balance in getting the proper nutrients from all the food groups. It will keep you from getting bored and giving up.

These lists may seem a bit overwhelming. Pick one or two you will incorporate and record it on page 49 in your journal. Try a few at a time and build in as many in as you can over time.

As you travel on your weight-loss journey, you will incorporate these into your new healthy lifestyle.

Bon appetit!

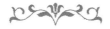

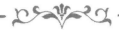

ENDNOTES

Chapter 1: How Did We Get This Way?

1. Cohen, R. "Sugar Love (A Not So Sweet Story)." *National Geographic Magazine*. August, 2013. Accessed April 9, 2016. ngm.nationalgeographic.com/2013/08/sugar/cohen-text

2. Peirce Thompson, Susan. "BHAG." Accessed April 9, 2016. http://susanpeircethompson.com/bhag/

3. West Virginia Department of Health and Human Resources. "Obesity: Facts, Figures , Guidelines: Obesity and Mortality." Accessed April 9, 2016. https://www.wvdhhr.org/bph/oehp/obesity/mortality.htm

4. West Virginia Department of Health and Human Resources. "Obesity: Facts, Figures, Guidelines: Executive Summary." Accessed April 9, 2016. https://www.wvdhhr.org/bph/oehp/obesity/execsum.htm

Chapter 2: Am I Really a Food Addict? Here's How to Tell

1. American Psychiatric Association. *Diagnostic and Statistical Manual of Mental Disorders* , 5th ed. Arlington, VA: American Psychiatric Publishing, 2013.

Chapter 3: Consequences of Our Love of Food

1. West Virginia Department of Health and Human Resources. "Obesity: Facts, Figures, Guidelines: Executive Summary." Accessed April 9, 2016. https://www.wvdhhr.org/bph/oehp/obesity/execsum .htm

Chapter 4: No More Excuses!

1. Rationalize. *Webster's Ninth New Collegiate Dictionary*. Springfield, MA: Merriam-Webster Inc., Publishers, 1984.

2. Desensitize. *Webster's Ninth New Collegiate Dictionary*. Springfield, MA: Merriam-Webster Inc., Publishers, 1984.

3. Svartefoss, Claudia. *Positively Perfect*. Amazon Digital Services LLC, 2015.

4. Sensitize. Webster's Ninth New Collegiate Dictionary. Springfield, MA: Merriam-Webster Inc., Publishers, 1984.

Chapter 5: What Are My Pain Points? How Do They Affect My Self Concept?

1. Casteix, Joelle. *The Power of Responsibility*. The Worthy Adversary Press, 2015.

2. Schema. *Webster's Ninth New Collegiate Dictionary*. Springfield, MA: Merriam-Webster Inc., Publishers, 1984.

3. Thomson, James: *The Formula for Christian Self Esteem*. Counselor's Heart Publishing, 2015.

Chapter 6: Where Does My Change Begin?

1. Casteix, Joelle. *The Power of Responsibility*. The Worthy Adversary Press, 2015.

2. Sorensen, Marilyn J. *Breaking the Chain of Low Self Esteem*, 2nd ed. Sherwood, OR: Wolf Publishing Co., 2006.

3. Elrod, Hal. *The Miracle Morning: The Not-So-Obvious Secret Guaranteed to Transform Your Life (Before 8 AM)*. Hal Elrod International, Inc., 2014.

4. Minchinton, Jerry. *Maximum Self-Esteem: The Handbook for Reclaiming Your Sense of Self-Worth*. Vanzant, MO: Arnford House Publishers, 1993.

Chapter 7: "Stinkin' Thinkin'" (Cognitive Distortions)

1. Burns, David D. *The Feeling Good Handbook: The New Mood Therapy*, Rev. ed. New York: Penguin Putnam Inc., 1999.

Chapter 8: Creating My New Identity

1. Irwin, Nancy B. "Mirror, Mirror on the Brain." *You Turn* (blog), June 4, 2011. Accessed April 9, 2016. https://drnancyirwin.wordpress.com.

2. Visualization. Webster's Ninth New Collegiate Dictionary. Springfield, MA: Merriam-Webster Inc., Publishers, 1984.

3. Casteix, Joelle. *The Power of Responsibility*. The Worthy Adversary Press, 2015.

4. Schwartz, Sara. "7 Surprising, Immediate Benefits of Exercise." Accessed April 17, 2016. www.grandparents.com/health-and-wellbeing/exercise-and-de-stress/immediate-benefits-of-exercise

Chapter 10: Danger Ahead: Watch Out for Sabotage!

1. Sorensen, Marilyn J. *Breaking the Chain of Low Self Esteem*, 2nd ed. Sherwood, OR: Wolf Publishing Co., 2006.

2. Delayed Gratification. Wikipedia. March 22, 2016. Accessed April 9, 2016. https://en.wikipedia.org/wiki/Delayed_gratification.

Chapter 11: Habits Will Make You or Break You!

1. "Habit Formation." *Psychology Today*. Accessed April 9, 2016. http://www.psychologytoday.com/basics/habit-formation.

2. Wood, W., & D. T. Neal. "A New Look at Habits and the Habit-Goal Interface." *Psychological Review* 114, no. 4:843-863. (2007). Accessed April 9, 2016. http://www.apa.org/pubs/journals/features/rev-1144843.pdf.

3. Bargh, J. A. "The Four Horsemen of Automaticity: Awareness, Intention, Efficiency, and Control in Social Cognition." In R. S. Wyer & T. K. Strull (Eds.), *Handbook of Social Cognition: Vol. I Basic Processes*, 1-40. Hove, England: Lawrence Erlbaum Associates Publishers, 1994.

4. Duhigg, Charles. *The Power or Habit: Why We Do What We Do in Life and Business.* New York, Random House, 2012.

Chapter 12: Accountability: It's Up to Me!

1. Daskal, Lolly. "Accountability: If It Is To Be, It's Up To Me." Lead From Within (blog), January 14, 2014.

Accessed April 9, 2016.
http://www.lollydaskal.com/leadership/accountabilit
y-if-it-is-to-be-its-up-to-me/

2. Bregman, Peter. "The Right Way to Hold People Accountable." *Harvard Business Review,* January 11, 2016. Accessed April 9, 2016. https://hbr.org/2016/01/the-right-way-to-hold-people-accountable#

Chapter 14: Stress—Do I Need a "Chill Pill"?

1. Burns, David D. *The Feeling Good Handbook: The New Mood Therapy*, Rev. ed. New York: Penguin Putnam Inc., 1999.

2. Greenberg, Melanie. "Why We Gain Weight When We're Stressed—And How Not To." *Psychology Today,* August 28, 2013. Accessed April 9, 2016. https://www.psychologytoday.com/blog/the-mindful-self-express/201308/why-we-gain-weight-when-we-re-stressed-and-how-not

3. Haden, Jeff. "9 Ways Reading Fiction Can Make You Happier and More Creative." Inc., November 19, 2015. Accessed April 9, 2016. www.inc.com/jeff-haden/9-ways-reading-fiction-can-make-you-happier-and-more-creative.html/

Chapter 15: Sleep, Glorious Sleep!

1. Lionel Bart. *Food Glorious Food.* Sydney, Australia: Essex Music, 1960.

2. Breus, Michael, J. "The Link Between Sleep and Weight Loss." *Huffington Post,* November 17, 2011. Accessed April 9, 2016. www.huffingtonpost.com/dr-michael-j-breus/sleep-weight-loss-and-appe_b_566378.html

3. Peirce Thompson, Susan. "BHAG." Accessed April 9, 2016. http://susanpeircethompson.com/bhag/

4. Ashton, Jen. "Sleep Deprivation and Your Weight." *Good Morning America*. November 2, 2015. Accessed April 9, 2016. http://abcnews.go.com/GMA/video/sleep-deprivation-effects-body-34909695

5. Crain, Esther. "The 11 Biggest Health Benefits of Sleep." *Huffington Post,* January 28, 2015. Accessed April 9, 2016. www.huffingtonpost.com/2015/02/38/biggest-sleep-health-bene_n_6549830.html

6. Sampson, Harold. "Psychological Effects of Deprivation of Dreaming Sleep." *The Journal of Nervous and Mental Disease* 143, no. 4:305–317 (October, 1966).

7. Hyman, Mark. "Sleep Tips: How to Sleep Better, Lose Weight, and Live Longer." *Huffington Post*, November 17, 2011. Accessed April 9, 2016. www.huffingtonpost.com/dr-mark-hyman/sleep-tips-how-to-sleep-b_416658.html

Chapter 16: Exercise—It Really ISN'T the "E" Word

1. Glanville, Nicola. "What Exercise Should I Do?" Accessed April 9, 2016. http://www.weightlossresources.co.uk/exercise/questions-answers/what-exercises-should-I-do.htm

2. Blackburn, Gordon. "What is the Best Type of Aerobic Exercise" Accessed April 9, 2016. https://my.clevelandclinic.org/

3. Mayo Clinic Staff. "Exercise: 7 Benefits of Regular Physical Activity." Healthy Lifestyle Fitness. Accessed April 16, 2016. www.mayoclinic.org/healthy-lifestyle/fitness/in-depth/exercise/art-20048389

4. Schwartz, Sara. "7 Surprising, Immediate Benefits of Exercise." Accessed April 9, 2016. www.grandparents.com/health-and-wellbeing/exercise-and-de-stress/immediate-benefits-of-exercise

5. Epiphaniou, Leoni. "What Happens to Your Brain When You Dance." ZLife (blog), September 5, 2015. Accessed April 9, 2016. https//www.facebook.com/zumba/posts/1029979133689425

6. Breene, Sophia, "13 Mental Health Benefits of Exercise." *Huffington Post,* March 27, 2013. Accessed April 9, 2016. www.huffingtonpost.com/2013/13/27/mental-health-benefits-exercise_n_2956099.html

Addendum: Other Guidelines to Consider

1. Zinczenko, David & Matt Goulding. 26 Bad Habits That Make You Fat. Eat This! Weight Loss (blog). Accessed April 9, 2016. www.eatthis.com/bad-habits-make-you-fat

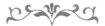

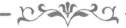

ABOUT THE AUTHOR

Wendy has been managing her weight successfully for the last 55 years. She has a passion for helping people (she is a licensed marriage and family therapist, practicing in San Marcos, California), and she cares about people who struggle with their weight. The birth of the idea for this book came from a friend who said, "Write whatever you're passionate about."

Having grown up in Boston and moving to Michigan as a teen, she attended Michigan State University and received her Bachelor of Arts in Music. In the mid-70s she was a secretary in the Middle East and evacuated to London after war broke out in Beirut. Upon returning to the United States, she worked in the courthouse in Colorado Springs and later at Hewlett-Packard.

Wendy met her husband, who was serving in the military, in Colorado Springs. They have four adult children. They are involved in Christian ministry and live in sunny Oceanside, California.

She enjoys reading, jigsaw puzzles, crossword puzzles, and baking, although she saves baking time for special occasions to avoid the collateral damage!

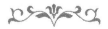

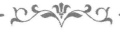

PLEASE!

Thank you for buying my book! I appreciate your feedback and love hearing what you have to say.

If you enjoyed reading this book and it was helpful to you, please leave a REVIEW on Amazon.com.

Thanks so much!!!

Wendy

If you would like further assistance in your weight-loss journey, check out my website at http://www.wendyhigdon.com, or you can reach me at wendy@wendyhigdon.com.

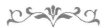

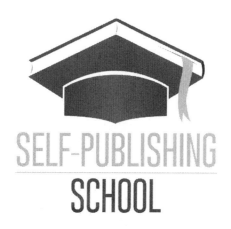

SELF-PUBLISHING
SCHOOL

NOW IT'S YOUR TURN

Discover the EXACT 3-step blueprint you need to become a bestselling author in 3 months.

Self-Publishing School helped me, and now I want them to help you with this FREE VIDEO SERIES!

Even if you're busy, bad at writing, or don't know where to start, you CAN write a bestseller and build your best life.

With tools and experience across a variety niches and professions, Self-Publishing School is the <u>only</u> resource you need to take your book to the finish line!

DON'T WAIT

Watch this FREE VIDEO SERIES now, and say
"YES" to becoming a bestseller:

http://bit.ly/wendy-sps

Made in the USA
San Bernardino, CA
08 January 2019